THE
FIRST NHS

THE FIRST NHS

HOW JOHN TOMLEY'S WORK LED TO MODERN HEALTHCARE

EMMA SNOW

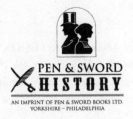

PEN & SWORD **HISTORY**

AN IMPRINT OF PEN & SWORD BOOKS LTD.
YORKSHIRE – PHILADELPHIA

First published in Great Britain in 2023 by
PEN AND SWORD HISTORY
An imprint of
Pen & Sword Books Ltd
Yorkshire – Philadelphia

ISBN 978 1 39903 816 4

Typeset in Times New Roman 11/13.5 by
SJmagic DESIGN SERVICES, India.
Printed and bound in the UK by CPI Group (UK) Ltd.

Pen & Sword Books Limited incorporates the imprints of Atlas, Archaeology,
Aviation, Discovery, Family History, Fiction, History, Maritime, Military,
Military Classics, Politics, Select, Transport, True Crime, Air World, Frontline
Publishing, Leo Cooper, Remember When, Seaforth Publishing, The Praetorian
Press, Wharncliffe Local History, Wharncliffe Transport, Wharncliffe True Crime
and White Owl.

For a complete list of Pen & Sword titles please contact
PEN & SWORD BOOKS LIMITED
George House, Units 12 & 13, Beevor Street, Off Pontefract Road,
Barnsley, South Yorkshire, S71 1HN, England
E-mail: enquiries@pen-and-sword.co.uk
Website: www.pen-and-sword.co.uk

or

PEN AND SWORD BOOKS
1950 Lawrence Rd, Havertown, PA 19083, USA
E-mail: uspen-and-sword@casematepublishers.com
Website: www.penandswordbooks.com

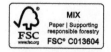

Contents

In season and out of season, on the public platform and in the Press, Bro. Tomley had been like a voice in the wilderness, crying out against the bad housing, bad nutrition and ravages of tuberculosis. He was trying to awake the conscience of his fellow men and eventually he won them over and the fiery cross was carried to the House of Commons.

– *Oddfellows Magazine, 1939.*

There is no subject that provides a wider field for discussion or arouses greater concern amongst those interested in the administration of the National Health Insurance Acts than the incidence of sickness among the insured population of the country. The matter is one of national importance, too, in its relation to the health and well-being of the community and its effect upon the economics of industry and even upon our national finances.

– *John Tomley, 'Tuberculosis and National Health Insurance', 1935.*

We are not facing a predestined plague, but a social problem, and we must work out our own salvation.

– *Jim Griffiths MP, debating the Welsh TB Inquiry report based on John Tomley's TB statistics in the House of Commons, 1939.[1] Griffiths later became minister for national insurance in 1945, working closely with Nye Bevan as minister of health and housing to set up the NHS and welfare state.*

[We recommend] an attack upon five giant evils: upon the physical Want with which it is directly concerned, upon Disease which often causes that Want and brings many other troubles in its train, upon Ignorance which no democracy can afford among its citizens, upon the Squalor which arises mainly through haphazard distribution of industry and population, and upon the Idleness which destroys wealth and corrupts men, whether they are well fed or not, when they are idle.[2]

– *William Beveridge, the Beveridge Report, 1942. Beveridge worked closely with Clement Davies MP, who had led the Welsh TB Inquiry.*

[The WNMA was] unique in its anticipation, so far as concerns broad outlines, of the pattern we have considered best for the future hospital service in general... I trust that the spirit of the Welsh National Memorial Association will live on and infuse vigour into the wider service upon which, with a feeling of high adventure, we are about to enter.[3]

– Nye Bevan, minister of health, writing to the WNMA board members including John Tomley, on the transfer of the first pilot national health service, the WNMA, to the NHS in 1948. The WNMA's headquarters at the Temple of Peace and Health in Cardiff became the headquarters of the NHS in Wales.

Preface

There's always been one branch of my family I didn't know much about as it was ravaged by a genetic disease and so passing on family history wasn't exactly our top priority. By the time I was a child, my granddad Edward couldn't speak and so, although I spent much of my early childhood in the same room as him, we never had a conversation. So, he never told me about his father, John Tomley. My mum was ill with the same disease from the time I was a teenager, so she couldn't gather her thoughts well enough to tell me either.

Then, in 2017, in the run-up to the seventieth anniversary year of the National Health Service, I passed by a stand at a conference and was asked, 'Were you or any of your relatives involved when the NHS was first set up, as the first patients or staff?' I dredged up something from the depths of my memory: twenty-five years before, aged 12, when I was helping my granny tidy her attic, she said to me, 'Your great-grandfather got a CBE for helping Nye Bevan set up the NHS.' At the time I had no idea what a CBE was, who Nye Bevan was, and only a hazy idea that the NHS was the local doctor's surgery and hospital. When I repeated this to the researcher, I replayed this in my head. A CBE?! Nye Bevan?! Setting up the NHS?! Now that I had spent most of my career working in health and social care, I knew exactly who Aneurin 'Nye' Bevan was, and suddenly realised this was actually rather important.

The researcher asked if I knew what role John Tomley played. I said he was a solicitor in a small town in Wales, so I suggested that perhaps he had helped with legal documents for the local doctor's surgery and hospital. I remembered my family said he had drafted legal… something or other. The researcher's response was that if he had got a CBE for his work, he must have played a national role. But what national role could he have possibly had from deep in the Welsh countryside, especially as Welsh people were hugely discriminated against at the time?

I remembered my granny also showed me some ribbons in a case which had belonged to John Tomley, saying they were from the Oddfellows, who she explained were 'like the Masons'. By the 1990s, all that we young people knew about the Masons was that they had funny handshakes. So that clearly wasn't relevant to the NHS. Or was it?

Over the next few years, I found out little pieces of information. The NHS seventieth anniversary had prompted the National Library of Wales to commission a report on how the work tackling tuberculosis (TB) in Wales led to the NHS being set up, and how John Tomley was one of the first public health statisticians. A few years later, I watched Ruth Jones' episode of *Who Do You Think You Are?*, which explained how the 'friendly societies' ran healthcare before the NHS – her father was a local leader in South Wales. So that explained why my granny had mentioned the Oddfellows – fraternal societies who ran the majority of healthcare and other services for working class people – when she told me about John's work setting up the NHS.

The biggest surprise was yet to come. More recently, I bought a subscription to look up historic newspaper articles online and was amazed to find the trail of articles mentioning John in the national press, explaining he represented the healthcare providers for 12 million workers and their families, so the majority of the country at the time, and covering his speeches. At our next family gathering, when I was telling my cousins about the articles and about my granny saying that John helped Nye Bevan set up the NHS, my uncle scoffed. 'No, it wasn't him helping Nye Bevan; the other way round, more like!'

Join me in my journey of discovery to finding out who my great-grandfather John Tomley actually was, and the pivotal role he played as a forefather of the NHS and welfare state. Not to mention the surprising contributions from other players who you might not know helped create the NHS and welfare state, including the Oddfellows, the Liberal Party, Winston Churchill, the *Daily Mirror* and even the Druids. This journey into the origins of the NHS and the welfare state will also give us all ideas for their future. How can we harness the same collaborative spirit and policy magic to work together today?

John was fired by indignation at the poor healthcare in the local workhouse in his small town in Wales. This inspired him to start the first ever national health service with MP David Davies, with the aim of eradicating TB in Wales, then collect national TB statistics for the first time and make the first business case for universal healthcare for TB patients, becoming one of the first public health statisticians. John was also one of the first local health commissioners, equivalent to the chief executive of an NHS Integrated Care Board today, where he piloted integrated health services. He went on to become the president of the National Conference of Friendly Societies, the largest part of the health service before it was the NHS, equivalent perhaps to the chief executive of the NHS today.

It turned out that John also got his CBE for setting up two, much earlier, national health services, rather than the 1948 NHS, although he was also a key player behind the 1948 version too. Those of us who work in the NHS today tend to think that the NHS was simply conceived by Nye Bevan in 1945 and sprang to life fully formed in less than three years after the Second World War. In fact, it was a very long gestation, with at least three pilots: the Welsh national TB service, and services during the First and Second World Wars. So, the NHS was at least the fourth national health service.

John had designed and set up the first ever national health service in the UK, for TB in Wales, in 1910, with David Davies. John then set up and ran a region of the second national health service, during the First World War, when hospitals had to work together to look after the large number of casualties. It turned out John hadn't drafted legal documents for the local hospital either – what my family had said was that he had drafted legislation. As a child I had not understood the difference. National legislation was far more important than the laws passed by MPs in the Houses of Parliament. John had got involved with this during the First World War.

John's policy and campaigning work based on his national TB statistics kicked off the Welsh TB inquiry in the 1930s. This then led directly to the Beveridge Report and the subsequent founding of the full NHS in 1948, which gained even more support when people saw the third national health service operating during the Second World War. The 'Five Giants', the evils facing society named in the Beveridge Report, were slain. Now everyone could enjoy healthcare, decent housing, employment or benefits to guarantee a minimum income for those unable to work, and education. Within a few years, TB mostly became a distant memory.

At the same time, John Tomley's foresight in campaigning for public health at national level and ensuring the foundation of the NHS and welfare state has had an enormous impact on us, his family. Unknown to John, every generation of his descendants would have a fatal genetic disease and need a lot of NHS care – including me. This has now come full circle, as NHS research has saved my daughter, John's great-great-granddaughter, the first generation to be born with a very low risk of the disease.

The NHS is still going strong, as Nye Bevan's supporters have often said, 'The NHS will last as long as there's folk with faith to fight for it'. Yet with recent cuts during austerity, followed by the effects of COVID, a lot of the prevention, self-management and home care services have been hugely cut, while NHS acute care has been protected from cuts as it is the most 'essential' service. This has led to people who would previously have been dealt with by other lower cost services having their conditions deteriorate and ending up in the longest ever queues of ambulances stuck outside A&E departments with 10-hour ambulance waits being common, and scathing newspaper headlines. How can John Tomley's wisdom in systems thinking and big data be rediscovered to help us today? How can we become the folk with faith to fight for the NHS?

Introduction

The Five Giants

'And I beheld a huge yellow-haired... man of vast size, and of horrid aspect, and a woman followed after him. And if the man was tall, twice as large as he was the woman... But thenceforth was there murmuring, because... they had begun to make themselves hated and to be disorderly in the land; committing outrages, and molesting and harassing... and thenceforward my people rose up and besought me to part with them...' said Matholwch unto Bendigeid Vran.

The Mabinogion[1]

The Mabinogion, the earliest stories of our island, dating from pre-Christian times, were written down in the *Red Book of Hergest* around 1400. They are in the pre-Saxon language which was used by the whole of England and Wales, and is now thought of as the Welsh language.

The dialogue quoted above is between Matholwch, king of Ireland, and Bendigeid Vran, the good giant and king of Britain (also known as Bran the Blessed), who accidentally let the evil giants into Britain. *The Mabinogion* is also the source of the tales of King Arthur and Merlin, or in Welsh Myrddin, the team who would fight off enemies like the evil giants.

As a student at Jesus College, Oxford University's college closely associated with Wales, I worked as a part-time librarian assigned to the college's Celtic Library, containing some of the oldest Welsh books in existence. I spent Sunday afternoons returning books to their shelves after use, and cleaning. Like something in a fairytale, the Celtic Library was narrow yet impossibly tall, with a huge ladder to reach the highest shelves and locked cupboards with the most valuable manuscripts. *The Red Book of Hergest* belongs to this collection, although fortunately now lives over in the Bodleian Library with professional librarians for safekeeping and not left up to students like me to dust.

Hanging precariously at the top of the ladder with one hand while dusting with the other, one day I considered my situation. My mum was ill but refused to admit it. She hadn't filled in the forms to get my student grant, and I already had the maximum student loan, so I had to work three jobs to get through my final year and graduate. I was being threatened with eviction by the college if I didn't pay my rent. I couldn't tell the college I was working the other jobs as it was against the rules for Oxford students to work during term time (aside from the few hours in the library) and I could be kicked out of college for it. Students couldn't claim benefits so there was no minimum income level for us. I was thankful that one of my other jobs, waitressing five nights per week at another college's canteen, gave me a free hot meal most days. A useful life lesson: waitresses never starve.

Yet all that was before we even reached the most difficult part – health, or rather, lack of it. I had to have a genetic test to find out if I was going to die young or not, if I wanted a child without my family's genetic disease. My mum had decided she didn't want to find out even though the rest of us already knew she was dying so I had been told by the doctor to keep my own test a secret from everyone apart from one friend. I was also my mum's main carer, yet she refused to move anywhere that I could get a job, and there were hardly any jobs in the part of Wales we came from. Certainly none where I could earn enough to support both of us. And I would have to leave my beloved boyfriend as there were no tech jobs for him there. People in Wales hadn't even heard of broadband. So our household income would be halved.

These troubles swirled dizzyingly around my head and I felt sick to the stomach from it all. Surely no one else had ever had this many problems at once? Shouldn't they just come one at a time?

I looked down for a safety net but there was none. Although other people enjoyed the safety net of the welfare state and a minimum income, I now saw there was a hole just below me that had been nibbled away. Despite the warm day, up that enormous ladder in that tall, cool stone room, I sensed a group of evil giants all breathing down my neck together, and I shivered.

The Mabinogion contains the story of how the evil giants got into Britain and caused havoc. Once the giants were out, they became numerous and prospered everywhere, and it was impossible to tackle the issue. Much like what is known as 'wicked' problems that face us as a society today, such as poverty, unemployment, health inequalities, homelessness. These issues so often hit people together, yet still come as a surprise for us. Take steps to eradicate an issue, and it unexpectedly comes back stronger, or changes and mutates into a different one.

Centuries later, such giants offered a very good metaphor for William Beveridge to choose for his report on what should be done to tackle these wicked problems, by suggesting starting the full NHS and welfare state.

In that 1942 report, *Social Insurance and Allied Services*, now generally known as the Beveridge Report, he wrote:

> The Plan for Social Security ... is one part only of an attack upon five giant evils: upon the physical Want with which it is directly concerned, upon Disease which often causes that Want and brings many other troubles in its train, upon Ignorance which no democracy can afford among its citizens, upon the Squalor which arises mainly through haphazard distribution of industry and population, and upon the Idleness which destroys wealth and corrupts men, whether they are well fed or not, when they are idle.[2]

These issues had been raised by the Welsh TB inquiry of 1937–1939, which I would learn was campaigned for by my great-grandfather John Tomley and was based on his statistics and other evidence. Did Beveridge know he was choosing a Welsh metaphor, I wonder, and was this intentional?

And who would be King Arthur and Merlin in this modern vision? David Davies, who had by then become Lord Davies, was more the establishment King Arthur figure, presiding over the national plan to eradicate TB in Wales and giving much of his gold to it. Like Arthur, his gold came from a cavern in the mountains too, the South Wales coal mines. By his side was policy and statistics wizard John Tomley, the Merlin in this tale.

Chapter 1

'Merits Rarely Combined'
1872–1905

John Tomley was born in the small town of Montgomery, mid Wales. His family lived in Clive House, a terraced black and white cottage on Chirbury Road. John's father, Robert Tomley, was born near Llanfair Caereinion, further into Wales, in 1834 to a Welsh family. John's mother, Esther Weaver, was born in 1844, the daughter of John Weaver, one of the hereditary freemen of Montgomery. Robert and Esther married in nearby Forden in 1872. They had two children, John in 1874 and his young sister Esther in 1876. At home with his family, John may have been known as Jack, a common nickname for people called John in those days.

John enjoyed an idyllic childhood in many ways.

Living in the countryside, the family's life was closely connected with the land and the seasons. The farms around them provided fresh milk, butter, cheese, eggs and meat. They grew fruit and vegetables in their garden. In this part of Wales, trees full of apples and damsons thrived. The children would forage blackberries on autumn walks through the fields and by the river, to be made into blackberry and apple crumble. Most gardeners grew potatoes, carrots and runner beans. When there was a glut of produce, it would be put into the cellar or made into jams and chutneys to keep healthy food available through the harsh winter. All this was supplemented by produce from local market gardeners sold in the grocer's shop and at the market at the town hall in Montgomery. Food that needed expensive greenhouses could be bought as a treat: cucumbers and tomatoes. Oranges and lemons were imported from Spain and eaten fresh or made into marmalade.

The countryside then was full of birds, animals, fish and insects. Footpaths criss-crossed the land, providing ways through the fields and down to the river for local workers and their families. John and his family could cross the low-lying yet very fertile 90 acres of Flos Lands, held in trust by the freemen of Montgomery. These were flooded each year by the river. John and his family could then wander along the banks of the River Camlad, just over a mile north from their home. The Camlad is the only river to flow from England into Wales, and it crosses the border twice before joining the River Severn.

Just before the Camlad joins flowing from the west, the Severn is joined by another of its major tributaries, the River Rhiew, flowing from the east. This is where I grew up, at Garthmyl, near the village of Berriew – in Welsh, Aberrhiew or 'mouth of the river Rhiew'. We lived in a canal workers' cottage which had been built with a lime kiln in the garden. In John's day, a century before, the kiln converted the materials coming in on canal boats to lime for farming and building. A small stream flowed down the side of the field by our house, an overflow from the canal controlled by what looked like a large metal ship's steering wheel which we longed to play with. When I was a toddler in a pushchair, my mum would walk me along the main road to a gap in the wall with railings. Peering through the railings, we could see where the stream from beside our house went into a larger lake, where my mum told me it was going into the River Severn. The other side was Montgomery, where our family came from, she said.

A mile or so to the east of John's home, the river was forded with stones, so that people, animals and carts could cross the river before the bridge was built. The ford was used in John's childhood, and was the main road to the rest of Wales, until about 1886. The river is rather large at this point, so the Welsh name for it, Rhyd Cwima, or 'the swift ford', is a warning. This ford was where the representatives of King Henry III and Llywelyn ap Gruffudd, the last Welsh Prince of Wales, met in 1267 to sign the Treaty of Montgomery, granting Wales a degree of autonomy. The village closest to the ford became, in English, Forden.

In John's day, Montgomery railway station arrived in 1861. Because of the rivers' geography, 'Montgomery' station was a mile or so away at Caerhowel and had missed Montgomery itself. Roads were quiet. No motor cars meant the only transport was a horse and cart, although, like John's family, few people could afford their own cart. Most people simply walked from place to place, as it was safe enough to walk on the roads, even for small children. John would have walked to primary school in Montgomery each day as a young child.

John enjoyed playing football and cricket at the nearby community pitches in the grounds of Lymore Hall, a crumbling yet picturesque Tudor half-timbered hunting lodge owned by the Earl of Powis. The Earl of Powis's main family home was nearby Powis Castle in Welshpool and the hunting lodge was surplus to requirements, so the building had not been maintained for many years. Yet Lymore Hall was still occasionally used by the earl for events, ranging from entertaining the Prince and Princess of Wales at a private shooting party to hosting the church bazaar with everyone in Montgomery invited.

At age 15, John joined the local men's cricket team for Montgomery which won 'very easily' against Bishop's Castle. Sidney Pryce, another of my great-grandfathers, was the captain.

John was also passionate about music. He sang in the chapel choir and learned to play the harmonium, a type of organ, and the flute. John's grandson, my uncle Chris Tomley, explained that before the days of television every home had to make their own entertainment and the majority had a piano and at least one person could play. For his organ lessons each week, John had to walk a six-mile round trip to Llandyssil, to get to his teacher.[1] John was dedicated to his playing and eventually was good enough to play the organ for his chapel.

John and his family attended the Calvinistic Methodist Chapel in Montgomery, which had been recently rebuilt with a schoolroom thanks to local fundraising. At one of the fundraising events when John was 11 years old, he met David Davies MP, a very successful local businessman who was a strict Calvinistic Methodist, and donated most of the money for the new building. Wales' first millionaire, he had worked his way up from nothing to become a railway builder and then coal mine owner. His company, Ocean Coal, was the largest in Wales, and supplied high quality steam coal for steamships and railways. He was the grandfather of the other David Davies MP who John would go on to work with.

At the new chapel schoolroom, there were lots of activities and events organised for teenagers. John played music and sang at concerts, was in a play of David and Goliath, and was involved in debates. As John got older, he became a youth leader and helped to organise summer treat outings for the younger children.

In those days, adults had to work within walking distance of home, in local farms or in their nearest town or village. John's father Robert worked close to home, splitting his time between Montgomery and Forden. Like many people, Robert may have moved to Montgomery as an adult because there were more jobs closer to the border of Wales. We know Robert had learned to read and write, as he worked as a clerk, so he had probably received schooling up to age 12 or 13. In those days, schools were mostly run by churches, charities and private individuals. He was on his way up in the world, along with his family. His better earnings as a clerk allowed him to send his son John to what we would now call secondary school from age 13 to 17, and these four years opened an even greater range of career opportunities for the young John.

There were no state secondary schools in that part of Wales at the time, so John travelled on the train to Kingsland School in Shrewsbury, across the border in England, near the former site of Captain Coram's Foundling Hospital and Shrewsbury's House of Industry – the local workhouse. Kingsland School was outside the town centre, on a hill overlooking the River Severn. A new principal, Welsh chapel minister Joseph Owen, had recently arrived from Machynlleth and had cannily started advertising in many Welsh language newspapers, encouraging Welsh-speaking parents to send their children to the nearest fully English-speaking town across the border so that they could do well in their careers, promising education for commerce, the professions and agriculture, a healthy situation, a 'good and liberal diet' and, most importantly for parents in Wales wanting to help their children go up in the world, low fees.[2]

John probably boarded in Shrewsbury to save on train fares. He did well there, particularly in maths. Principal Joseph Owen wrote in a later employment reference for him:

> His work evidenced three merits rarely combined in one pupil, namely the ability to unravel the intricacies of problems, very rapid solutions and correct results, even in exceptionally lengthened operations. I always considered that Mr Tomley would be just the man for any post requiring a quick and correct manipulation of figures.[3]

When John wasn't at school, he may have got involved in pranks with the other boys in Montgomery, a popular local pastime for teenagers in the days before television. These included blindfolding a friend and tying him to someone's door knocker, and twitching a thread with a button on to make a scraping noise at a window while standing some distance away. Let's hope John was never on the receiving end of the most dangerous local prank: tying up a boy and dropping him into the saw-pit at Lymore, leaving him to get out as best he could.[4] Chirbury Road, where John and his family lived, was known to be a rough area of the town and was famous for women's brawls, started by quarrelling neighbours.[5]

The giants are on the loose

During John's idyllic childhood, a visitor to Montgomery would be charmed by the rural life and the country sights. There was just one problem. The Five Giants stalked the land, with early death trailing in their wake. What Beveridge would come to call Idleness, Want, Disease, Ignorance and

Squalor in today's language would be Unemployment, Poverty, Disease, Ignorance and Homelessness.

The giants were related and often tossed their unfortunate victims from one giant to the next. From Unemployment came Poverty, and from Poverty came Disease, for example. Or from Disease came inability to work and then Unemployment. Once the giants had chosen their victim, it was nearly impossible to escape their clutches.

How could people fall into poverty? There were so many ways. The world was set up on three key assumptions: all men would work to provide for their families, work would be available which would pay enough to feed their families, and all women and children would be reliant on their menfolk.

There were just a few issues with this. Often, work was not available for men, or the work which was available did not pay enough. In many cases too, the man got sick, was injured or died, and was not able to provide for his family. Sometimes the stress of providing was too much and the man left, too. Widowed women could remarry, but they might no longer have their looks to attract a new partner, and often came with the burden of existing children. Many widows became desperate and lowered their standards, not to just to unattractive men, but also to controlling or violent men. Children were then at risk from their new stepfathers. Older children might feel forced to leave home, even if they had nowhere to go.

The Forden Workhouse

There were few refuges from the Five Giants in those days. Often the only place people could go was the workhouse. John's father Robert knew all about the Five Giants as he worked in the local workhouse in Montgomery and the surrounding area, based at Forden. A local poem from 1882 explains people's fear of the workhouse.

> Next perhaps a speech about Peace and Plenty,
> But, Oh, poor souls, your pocket's empty.
> Thus we toil on through life to Jordan;
> Let's hope that none may call at Forden!
> And in that red brick mansion stay
> Till death shall help them on their way![6]

Many residents died from malnourishment and disease, which spread rapidly in the confined spaces.

As a child, I remember driving along the road from my granny's house in Garthmyl. The Forden Institution, a huge red brick building, was a key landmark. To get to her best friend Trudy's home, we had to turn right at the Institution. 'That's the Institution!' my granny would exclaim. She often explained that it had been the workhouse and then a mental hospital. We had seen the musical *Oliver!*, so we thought workhouses were only run by bad people. We had no idea that, up until the NHS was established in 1948, workhouses were in fact the only place poor people could access healthcare if they couldn't afford to pay, and were often run by dedicated staff who wanted to support people who had fallen on hard times as best they could, despite huge underfunding. I don't recall her mentioning that her father-in-law John Tomley and his father Robert ran the workhouse. Yet they also fought to close it for good. It was perhaps a bit too complicated for children to understand.

Montgomery was the county town for the whole area, Montgomeryshire, which is now part of Powys, the county spanning from north to south Wales along the border with England marked by Offa's Dyke and the Welsh Marches. An area fought over by Marcher Lords and Welsh Princes, full of earthworks and castles. As John himself put it: 'Stirring is the story these ruined walls could tell of the Border contests which waged around this historic hill through the centuries of strife for the mastery of Wales.'[7]

Montgomery Castle, right on the border, was built by William the Conqueror's henchman Roger de Montgomery to control the Welsh. A few years after the Norman invasion, the conquerors had yet to get the people in order. Roger's son Robert of Belleme rebelled against William II and so Montgomery Castle was given to Baldwin de Boulers instead. The town around the castle became 'the town of Baldwin' – in Welsh, Trefaldwyn. In English, the name Montgomery persisted. And so the town ended up with two different names in the two different languages spoken by its people.

The historic Welsh/English split still echoes in the community today and would have been very much alive in Robert and John Tomley's time. Wales remained the first colony of England. While people in England did not necessarily mean to control the Welsh, the effect of a shared parliament where the majority of MPs were English and a majority vote was needed to make any decisions meant that anything which only affected Wales, or where Wales was being treated unfairly, could not be tackled by the Welsh MPs. So the relationship between the two communities remained one of the colonising English and colonised Welsh. Welsh people, like colonised people everywhere, recast our story so that we felt we had the cultural capital, even though we had effectively no legal power. To the Welsh, the English were in charge but boring. The Welsh were the rebels, Israelites in Egypt, persecuted by the English. Children of warrior spirit and song, with our true intentions disguised from the English by using our own language.

In those days, the majority of people only spoke Welsh. In 1847, when Robert was 13, education in Wales and in the Welsh language was condemned by senior English government reviewers. Welsh-speaking children struggled to learn in English-only schools with English textbooks. The reviewers, who only spoke English, had no experience of Wales or educating working-class children, and were prejudiced against the Welsh, were guided by Anglican ministers who were jealous of the success of the nonconformist and Welsh-speaking churches.

Yet the review had well-meaning origins. It had been suggested by a Welsh-born MP for an English constituency who hoped that Welsh people could be supported to learn English so that more jobs would be available to them in England. Traditional farming jobs were drying up and protests had started among working people across England and Wales. This sounded like a useful topic. So, what went wrong?

The lead reviewer was very young and inexperienced. He seems to have been prejudiced partly as a result of not having met Welsh people before. He and his fellow reviewers did not speak Welsh and were not even educationalists. Then, rather than sticking to his given topic of how more people could learn English, he widened his remit into a study of the morals of Welsh people.

Rather than considering the introduction of Welsh-medium schools with Welsh textbooks, the reviewers concluded that the nonconformist churches were holding back education by allowing the use of Welsh. People who spoke Welsh were more likely to be poor, dirty, lazy, ignorant and immoral. That these issues stemmed from poverty, and in fact were similar to the situation for poor people in England at the time, was not considered – it was clearly the Welsh language that was at fault. Therefore, Welsh should no longer be allowed in schools – it was made a moral issue. This so-called 'Treachery of the Blue Books' – the resulting report by the English reviewers – decimated the use of the Welsh language. Children were beaten if they spoke Welsh – this continued up to the 1930s and 40s. Robert's generation was therefore likely the last in the family to speak Welsh regularly and he would have ensured that his son John was brought up speaking English as his mother tongue, to avoid punishment at school and give him the opportunity of a career in an anti-Welsh atmosphere.

By Robert's day, in the early nineteenth century, Montgomery was still an important county town, but other towns in Montgomeryshire with more central train stations were growing larger, particularly Newtown.

In Newtown, local entrepreneur Pryce Pryce-Jones had set up the first ever mail-order firm, the Amazon of its day, in 1861. In 1879, when Robert's son John was five, Pryce-Jones built the huge red brick Royal Welsh Warehouse opposite Newtown train station, sending out woollen goods via the new railway to customers ranging from the Russian army, who bought sleeping bags, to Florence Nightingale and Queen Victoria, who favoured his wool flannel underwear. Business was thriving in Newtown for local people living close by and those lucky enough to land jobs there.

Yet for people living further out in the countryside around Montgomery, agricultural labourers who were gradually losing their farm jobs to mechanisation, times were tough. There was no safety net for unemployed people like there is today. If you lost your job or became too ill to work, tough. You would lose your home and your family would starve.

The only ray of hope for people in these dire situations was the local Poor Law relief. The local parishes, later local authorities, had a system where charity aid was given to those in most need. From the Elizabethan Poor Law in 1601 until the 1830s, this was mostly in the form of 'outdoor relief', where people on low incomes were given money, food, clothing or other goods. It wasn't generous, yet there was the prospect of keeping a modest home together and staying with your family.

In 1815, the Napoleonic Wars came to a close, ending a source of income for many young men. By 1830, after three successive bad harvests, there was mass unemployment across the UK. The Poor Law relief was overstretched and could not cope with the level of need. To better prioritise the worst-off people, it was decided to move to a system of 'indoor relief' or workhouses. If you wanted support, you now had to go into the workhouse, a cruel regime with harsh punishments for the slightest misdemeanour, where parents were separated from children and made to work all day at menial tasks such as breaking stones or picking oakum, in order to pay for their board and lodgings. This was meant to be off-putting to all but the very poorest people who had no choice. In the Forden workhouse, children aged 10 and over had to plait straw for hats and bonnets. Men were made to do harsh stone-breaking work, making smaller stones for road building, which were then sold to the local councils.

Fortunately, Charles Dickens' 1838 novel *Oliver Twist*, showing the worst of workhouse life, became very popular, and there was growing public support to improve the workhouse system. Yet this still took many decades to accomplish.

Robert Tomley was the first of the Tomleys to be involved in running the local workhouse. He is first shown on the 1871 census, aged 37 and single, with the occupation of relieving officer for Montgomery. This meant he was the Montgomery town council staff member who managed giving out Poor Law relief in the Montgomery area, primarily at the Forden Union workhouse.

The Forden Union was the new workhouse body established in 1870 to replace the much-hated Montgomery and Pool Union, which ran the Forden workhouse up to that date. It sounds like Robert was fortunate that he was working with rather more enlightened people. In 1870, the *Montgomeryshire Express* reported a change in policy: 'The Forden Board of Guardians – a body which does not as a rule act upon the side of generosity – has decided to purchase footballs, cricketing tack, skipping ropes, etc, for the use of the children in the workhouse.'

We next hear of Robert Tomley in the newspaper in 1880. The Montgomery Petty Sessions report states that a labourer has been called to the court to explain why he was not contributing financially to support his mother and father, who were receiving four shillings per week from the Forden board of guardians, represented by Robert as relieving officer. Their address is given as 'the Cliffe' which suggests this is outdoor relief – the parents were living in their own home and had not been forced to move into the workhouse yet. The labourer's wife gave evidence that her husband did not have regular work, and they had four children to support. The case was dismissed, so the labourer's family were not forced to pay to support their parents – perhaps better treatment than people would have received at earlier times and evidence of a change against the idea that the family should always pay.

Three great-grandfathers fighting the Five Giants

As well as my great-great-grandfather Robert Tomley, in the next generation his son John and two of my other great-grandfathers, Dr Ray Snow and Sidney Pryce, were all involved in running the local workhouses. Of course, they didn't know that their children and grandchildren would marry then. They just knew each other as colleagues and friends in Montgomery and the surrounding area.

Dr Ray Snow was the eldest, born in 1847. Ray was the doctor in Caersws, a small village the other side of Newtown, and the next railway station after

Newtown. As with most GPs in those days, his surgery in Severn Villas, Caersws, was also his home. An arched alleyway down the side led to the surgery room and dispensary. As well as being the GP, Ray also looked after sick people in Caersws Workhouse and others in the surrounding areas. Despite newspaper reports praising his talents early in his career, and high-profile patients including David Davies at Plas Dinam, as an Irish doctor he faced a lot of discrimination.

Ray was the medical officer for the local Llandinam Friendly Society, equivalent to a GP for the society members who were working people. They wrote Ray a reference explaining that he had been 'most assiduous and unremitting in his attention to all cases' and at all times treated people 'with uniform kindness and sympathy'. Another reference was signed by seventy-five farmers, businessmen and women in the local area, who Ray had treated. Thanks to these glowing recommendations, Ray was appointed as medical officer of health for Llanwnog District and Caersws Workhouse in 1891. The workhouse medical officer roles had been required for some time, yet the district posts were new. They had recently been introduced by local authorities and covered everyone in the local area, including homes and schools. Ray's job included vaccinations, inspections and making recommendations about isolation in cases of infectious disease. For example, in 1894 Ray closed Caersws Primary School after many cases of diphtheria over the Christmas holidays. In other years it was measles or scarlet fever. Vaccinations were a new way to prevent disease, and Ray organized vaccination clinics around the district, where local people could be vaccinated against smallpox free of charge.

The workhouse was a much riskier place to work. In those days, workhouses were full of TB, a deadly and untreatable disease, and doctors often succumbed to this themselves. Ray was lucky in that he avoided TB, yet he suffered a severe head injury when he was thrown from his horse when riding to a medical emergency in the countryside. The local paper reported he was in a coma for over a week.

Afterwards, Ray continued to work but was never the same, finding it more difficult to travel to his workhouse duties and emergency home visits, and slurring his words. The local paper reported the workhouse board of guardians criticizing him for not turning up to his workhouse role on time. Ray struggled to make enough money to feed his nine children. At the same time, he was kind-hearted about his patients, and often did not press for payment if people could not afford it. His son Jack remembered him spending money on red flannel petticoats which he gave to his poorer women patients living remotely in the hills around his practice. This was a form of preventative medicine to ward off illness and save him visits during the busiest winter months.

Sidney Pryce was fifteen years younger than Ray. He grew up in Kerry, the son of the pub landlord, so he knew Ray as a local doctor.

As a boy, Sidney loved practical jokes: pretending to be injured with pig's blood; hiding a neighbour's prize pig in the village hearse; hauling the village carrier's cart to the top of a tree with ropes; and attaching a drunken pub customer's horse and trap to a gate, so that he couldn't work out why the vehicle wasn't moving.[8]

Yet despite Sidney's joking about, he had a tragic family story. The youngest son, Sidney was the only one of Robert Pryce's four sons to survive to old age; the others all died sad or odd deaths. Local people said that it was because the family lived in a haunted house where a murder had previously taken place.

Sidney then moved to Montgomery, qualified as a solicitor, and started his own law firm. Sidney's work included acting as the clerk for the local workhouse and the local council. He was clearly keen to help people in need because he got involved with the workhouse. He also seems, from the minutes in the local paper, to have been a jolly figure, laughing and joking and generally smoothing over relationships when meeting attendees became fractious.

John starts work

John Tomley became my third great-grandfather to be involved in running the local workhouses. After secondary school, in 1891, 17-year-old John applied for a job in Montgomery, and started work as a solicitor's clerk at a law firm on Arthur Street. His new employer was Sidney Pryce, my other great-grandfather, by then a 29-year-old local solicitor. Sidney sponsored John to train as a solicitor too.

John and Sidney already knew each other well from having been on the same cricket team for two years. Sidney was captain of the Montgomery Cricket Club and John had joined the team a couple of years earlier.

As a clerk, John would have had to attend meetings, make notes, write up documents and fill in forms. John's work for Sidney included three different roles, so it was quite a lot to take in. Fortunately, John was a fast learner.

First, John had to help Sidney with the normal legal work of the solicitors firm: helping people with house sales, court cases and so on. John had to arrange client meetings and then attend them with Sidney, finding the right files and taking notes in each meeting. Over time, as John went through his solicitor's training, he could take on more complex parts of the work and do more by himself, with Sidney checking.

Sometimes the meeting would be at Sidney's office. Other times, they might have to travel further away to meet the client, at their office, farm or home. A lot of clients were older people writing their wills or needing support managing their affairs because of illness. Sometimes this could lead to unexpected outcomes: Sidney was once chased with a gun by a client who had mistaken him for a relative he had fallen out with, and had to escape by running down the railway line.

John's second job was to help Sidney with his role as clerk to the board of guardians of Forden Workhouse. The board of guardians was the group of people who made all the important decisions about running the workhouse – like a board of governors – often including people considered 'the great and the good'. Typically, this was well-off people who had more time on their hands. In those days, rich people were thought to be better at running things, although this was more a matter of being lucky enough to be born into a rich family who could afford to educate their children well. Poor people had much less education so many people would have struggled to even read the meeting papers. Only rich men could vote, too, so they were the only people with political influence over MPs and local councils, who had the clout to get things done.

The board of guardians would have met every month or two, with paid staff running the workhouse in between times. John became the assistant clerk for the workhouse, arranging meetings, putting together meeting papers for discussion, attending the meetings with Sidney, taking minutes of the decisions made in the meeting, and writing up the notes. John's father Robert worked at the workhouse part time, and often came to the meetings to report on progress with his work, as well as sending in written reports to the board of guardians.

The third job John had to do was to help Sidney with his role as clerk to Montgomery Town Council. This was the local authority, similar to local councils everywhere these days, except that the area covered by each council was a lot smaller. Councils today look after perhaps 200,000 people. In those days, it might have only been 2,000. This meant each area only had a very small budget and part-time staff, like John and Sidney. John's father Robert also worked at the council part time.

The councillors met every month or so, and John's role for the meetings was similar to that at the workhouse. He became the finance clerk, so he would also have had to collect all the bills that needed paying, arrange for them to be paid, then write a report on spending. This was funded by people paying rates – what today we know as business rates and council tax. From time to time, when the amount of rates that people should pay was being decided, John had to calculate the amount of money that each taxpayer needed to contribute to fund the council's overall costs. John also had to deal with the auditors, the people reviewing the council's accounts and bills, to check everything had been accounted for correctly. This was no mean feat for a 17-year-old who was a trainee solicitor, not a trainee accountant. Surprisingly, for many years after businesses and charities required qualified accountants as finance directors, the public sector didn't. The public sector requirement was only introduced about fifteen years ago, a few years after I qualified as an accountant myself.

Romance and entertainment

Life wasn't all work and no play for John at this time though. John's cricket playing improved quickly under his employer Sidney Pryce's captaining: the next year, in a match against Machynlleth, Sidney scored the most runs of the match, 47, with John second at 25 runs. In another match that summer, John managed to turn the tables and score more runs than Sidney for the first time. Sidney introduced John to social events like the cricket club dinner at a local pub, where there was much raucous singing. The year after, there was a tribute to John in the speeches: 'defeat stared them in the face, but the plucky play of a young batsman, Mr J.E. Tomley, turned the tables and secured for them a brilliant victory.'[9]

John also made friends with Robert Bunner, a young man a couple of years older, who was starting a hardware shop next door to John's new workplace on Arthur Street. Robert wasn't the only young person on Arthur Street. John also became friends with Edith Soley, almost literally the girl next door. She lived above her father's grocery and baker's.

Edith's father, Thomas Soley JP, was the son of a Thomas Soley who had emigrated to America. Thomas junior then came back twelve years later, and took over his grandfather George's grocery shop in Montgomery.

Edith and John had met at chapel. Edith's father, Thomas, was one of the chapel leaders and probably rather strict, in line with chapel traditions laid down by his own preacher grandfather George, who had been a Calvinistic Methodist preacher as well as a grocer. Now it fell to John to work out how to woo Edith in a way which her father would approve of. John had a brainwave – he wrote to the principal of Bala Theological College to ask whether dancing was appropriate for young people who went to chapel, and got it published in the paper. Fortunately, the answer was that dancing should be allowed as long as there were respectable older people there to supervise it, and there were 'no intoxicating drinks'.[10]

As well as indoor dances, there was another, more rebellious, opportunity to dance at Montgomery in those days. Dancing on the old castle ruins was organised by young people themselves and does not sound like it involved much adult supervision. Old Mrs Mostyn recalled that when she was young, they would dance on the castle with music: Mr Marshall, the Post Office, had an English Concertina, Dick Proctor played the 'cello and Reuben Maddox played the fife.[11]

The first event we hear of in the newspaper with John and his future wife Edith was at a Cricket Club fundraising concert in 1891. Did John manage to speak to Edith, or did they just exchange looks across a crowded room? The article mentions 'the elite' gracing Montgomery with their presence for this event – a group of the very rich, including Sir Pryce Pryce-Jones – the local mail order millionaire – and a number of MPs, who at that time would have been all rich people too, because only property-owning men could vote. This meant no one of middle and lower incomes was represented, a situation that the Liberal Party were working to improve. By 'improve' this meant, at the time, a partial improvement so that other men who owned small amounts of property could vote. The idea of all adults voting, including women, would have to wait another 40 years. This shows the forelock-tugging world John was born into, reliant on persuading the toffs to make a charitable contribution to fulfil any health, education or social needs in the local community; and it would later be the visionary power of his generation to imagine a better world and make it happen.

There was romance in the air for 29-year-old Sidney Pryce too. John's boss was interested in one of the Newill sisters, 24-year-old Mary Medlicott Newill. Her sister Ethel, a year older, sang several songs including a duet with the vicar and two solos. The Newills were an extremely musical family.

By March 1892, John had managed to get a little closer to Edith – they were both in a show together at the Mutual Improvement Society Social Evening. John sang a comic song, 'Poor Married Man', before playing the flute in the slightly misnamed Amateur String Band, both performances being encored. This time, John's future wife Edith was performing too, playing the opening piece of a piano duet, 'The Sleigh Race'.

Oddfellows Lodge 50th Jubilee

On 23 June 1891 John attended his first local Oddfellows lodge meeting. The Oddfellows fraternal societies had their origins in the early 1700s and by this time had spread across Britain in various branches. Robert Tomley, John's father, was already an active member. Robert had moved to Montgomery from Llanfair, where he had been active in another local friendly society there, the Sons of Gomer Society. On moving to Montgomery, Robert first acted as secretary of the local lodge of Oddfellows. After that, he became treasurer, then the lodge leader, known as 'Noble Grand', and then a trustee. As a former lodge leader, he was then called 'Past Grand'. So Robert was keen to encourage his son John to follow in his footsteps by joining the movement.

The full name of the Montgomery lodge was the Montgomery Loyal Ark of Friendship Lodge of Oddfellows. Lodges were the local branches of the organisation, run by local members themselves. All Oddfellows lodges had unique names in order to tell them apart, and in order to inspire local people.

John would later speak about the meaning of the name when the lodge had been set up in the 1840s: '... there was great agitation as to the condition of employment and of the working classes, and the Chartists were in existence. At the same time, there was an undercurrent of thrift and self-reliance, and it was that which led to the formation of the friendly societies... "Ark" meant refuge, and the lodge was a refuge for those who were in times of difficulty.'[12]

John's first meeting was a special event, the lodge's golden jubilee celebration. In the morning, all the members and their children met at the lodge's meeting room and formed a procession headed by the Newtown Brass and Reed Band. Brass bands were a key part of the working men's movement, as the musicians could walk along and play at the same time, so they were ideal for parades and political demonstrations. The members and officers had special regalia to wear, showing their status. An illuminated banner combined to make what the local paper called 'a most effective display'.

After a parade around the town, the Oddfellows marched to Lymore Park, the local stately home, where the owner, the Earl of Powis, had allowed a tent to be put up. A local pub, the Gullet Inn, had provided lunch for everyone, and this was followed by speeches.

John's boss, Sidney Pryce, was also an Oddfellows member and made a speech: 'From statistics which he had before him, he found that the funds of the society amounted to £7,000,000, and the number of members present was 700,000 (applause). Those figures spoke well for the society, and it was also well worthy of notice that during the last year, several Acts of Parliament had been passed for the support of such societies, and the advancement of the interests which they promoted.' In today's terms, the £10 funds saved up per member to help them out in times of trouble would be equivalent to £1,400 per member today – a useful sum to tide people over temporarily for a month or two, yet not enough to fund hospital treatment or retirement.

John's father, Robert, also spoke, expressing his pleasure that younger men were joining the society – no doubt a hint to John and his friends. The newspaper report of his speech said: 'During the year 1890, £233 9s 7d was paid in sick pay, and since the beginning of 1891, £103 had been paid out in that way… However they were fortunate in having plenty of money at their backs – (hear, hear) – so that when a time of excessive sickness came they were able to meet it.' This payout was likely due to the huge worldwide respiratory virus pandemic of 1889-90 known as 'Asiatic flu'.

Now that the boring bit was over, young John and his friends could enjoy themselves for the rest of the day. Sidney and John helped organise the sports, an 'excellent programme of athletic contests and pony races' with 'a large number of spectators'. The band played throughout the afternoon, at intervals, for dancing. At 10 pm, a dance was held in the Town Hall, with music provided by a quadrille band.[13]

How fantastic to find John's father Robert stating his fervent hope to 17-year-old John and his generation that they would work hard to continue the friendly society work and hopefully celebrate the centenary in 1941 'under as favourable and auspicious circumstances'. John did live this long and would by that time have led the whole friendly society moment nationally, and the momentum for welfare provision he would inspire certainly led to even more favourable and auspicious circumstances than I am sure Robert and his generation could have envisaged in 1891.

Brother Tomley

At the time, there was really only one way for working people to ensure at least minimal healthcare was available to them. This was through the friendly societies, which were originally founded for working people to contribute money in good times and then use collective healthcare in bad times – effectively a form of insurance policy. In this way, if you were unlucky enough to be sick a lot, you shared your risk with other people who were more able to work.

When the earliest friendly societies were set up from 1810 onwards, the ruling classes were so rattled that they moved to outlaw them. No way should the working men band together! While this seems unbelievable to us, given that the friendly societies were merely about things like sharing the cost of a doctor, an innocent enough purpose, there was concern about what this might lead to. In fact, the friendly societies did lead to what the ruling classes most feared – workers banding together for health, then education, then forming the labour movement, then the election of the Labour Party, which finally implemented the NHS over a century later. Worker education made it possible for working people to develop the skills needed to operate as union organisers, councillors and finally, MPs.

The early outlawing of the friendly societies meant that they had to operate underground. The secret handshakes might seem silly to us now, yet were incredibly important at this time. They showed who was a genuine member and who it was safe to talk to. In the days before most workers could write, these secret handshakes also provided a form of secure identification and fraud prevention, showing they were entitled to the medical benefits as they had contributed to the pot.[14],[15]

Over time, the friendly societies were legally allowed to operate again. As the new Poor Law policy hit after 1830, replacing outdoor relief with only indoor relief at the workhouses, disease shot up even more because of many people being kept in close quarters with other families at the workhouses. A workhouse policy was to split up families, meaning people were transferred between workhouses, spreading disease further afield. Workers were more in need of collective medical benefits than ever, to prevent the threat of the workhouse for their families. Membership of the friendly societies shot up and by the late 1930s there would be over 12 million members.

Friendly societies started off just providing medical benefits for the main earner in the family, which at the time meant men of working age. The other members of the family – women, children and retired people – did not get a look-in, apart from an occasional grant for maternity, to pay for a midwife or doctor to attend a birth. This was because everyone was reliant on the working men as the breadwinners for the whole family; if there was a choice to be made, their healthcare had to come first. At the start, there simply wasn't enough money to provide for the rest of the family. Over time, the argument was successfully made by John Tomley and others to extend healthcare to the rest of the family, especially in the case of communicable diseases such as TB.

The amount of healthcare provided by friendly societies was also limited by the amount working men could reasonably contribute. A family doctor was usually the most it could run to – there was no thought of hospital treatment.

The first hospitals were charities and mostly had rich patients who subsidised the odd poorer person having treatment there. There were a lot more poor people than rich people, so the amount that could be subsidised was very limited. Over time, the friendly societies set up their own hospitals and sanatoriums for the treatment of TB and other diseases, aided by John Tomley and others, and funded by benefactors including Lord Davies.

So why did my granny show me the Manchester Unity of Oddfellows ribbons that John Tomley had owned? The mystery is solved – the Oddfellows were a friendly society, and therefore ran healthcare. At the time the Manchester Unity of Oddfellows was the biggest friendly society in the UK, covering many different areas including John's home town of Montgomery in mid Wales.

While Robert and John worked in the workhouse by day and saw the horrors there, in the evening they could encourage working people to join the friendly society in order to avoid the workhouse. The friendly societies called all their members 'Brother', in order to show that everyone was equal. John therefore became Brother John, and the papers report from then on all of his friendly society work as 'Bro. Tomley…'.

Many other friendly societies existed at the time too. By the late 1800s there were around 27,000 registered friendly societies in the UK. Many of the friendly societies set up and incubated new ones. I currently spend part of my week working in the former Great Western Railway Hospital, which is now a community centre. This complex was named by Nye Bevan as a birthplace of the NHS. The GWR railway workers were inspired by the Oddfellows who had helped found an educational institute next door, and organized their own friendly society, the GWR Medical Fund. This was one of the first to offer hospital care to working people and to insure unemployed people with the contributions of employed people, a key factor in later National Insurance.

First council meeting, the suffragettes and the press

On 3 November 1891, John attended Montgomery Town Council as the finance clerk, assisting his employer, Sidney Pryce. This was John's first local government meeting and much of the discussion and jargon must have gone over his head to start with. I can imagine a 17-year-old trying desperately not to yawn during a long discussion on 'A Point of Municipal Law' and waiting for his section at the end, to present the bills needing to be paid.[16] Yet John had to get to grips with the art of administration in order for him to achieve so much later in life.

Little could the older men at the meeting know that this new 17-year-old trainee would one day cause their entire council to be abolished, amalgamated into a much larger unit of local government in order to better achieve public health, housing and education aims as part of the welfare state. What would they have made of that, I wonder?

A little more interest for John may have been given by being able to meet George Farmer, one of the councillors mentioned at the meeting, who is another family member on my dad's side. Dr Ray Snow, my other great-grandfather, had married George's niece Edith Farmer. At this time, George would have lived at The Hollies in Montgomery, the house John himself later lived in.

As George's great-nephew Angus Snow, my uncle, put it:

> George lived there with Edith's four unconventional cousins... George had a son and three daughters. Richard became a solicitor and Recorder for Chester. Alice [aged 24 in 1891] was one of the first women to gain a degree at Somerville College, Oxford, in 1909. Later, Rosa [aged 27 in 1891] and Ada [29] were to join her in the suffragette movement.
>
> Alice chained herself to Buckingham Palace railings and did time in Holloway Prison for it where she went on hunger strike and was force-fed. She received one of the medals that Mrs Pankhurst had cast for those in Holloway Prison. It is now owned by Mrs Joyce Whitfield, of Criccieth, together with the hammer with which she broke Mr Asquith's window in Downing Street.[17]

How much was John inspired by these rebellious and glamorous local girls a few years older than him? Suddenly Welsh people from Montgomery, deep in the countryside, could change the world. John chose a pragmatic middle path between outright illegal rebellion and the unhelpful administrative strictures of the Victorian era that were holding back reforms to improve equality in society. Let's call it 'radical administration'.

Also in November, John was mentioned twice in the same newspaper column of the *Montgomeryshire Express*. He had also become the correspondent for Montgomery, and all 'Orders for Advertisements and Notices of Meetings' should be sent to him, giving him an important connection to local communications at a time when newspapers were the only mass media.

First committee roles

Outside work, John started to take on volunteer roles on committees. Still aged 17, he also joined the Band of Hope committee (a Christian temperance charity), along with his mother. Next, he helped set up a Mutual Improvement Society for young men, which met in the chapel schoolroom and included talks and debating. John won a debating prize there. A few months later, John and his debating friends travelled to the neighbouring village of Berriew, where I grew up. The annual team and competitive meeting was held in the Assembly Rooms, Efel Fach. John and a friend named Evans teamed up in a debating competition for 'Best Impromptu Discussion – Cricket or Football' and drew as joint winners with another team. It is interesting to see that John was sharpening his debating skills and powers of persuasion which he would put to great use later in life.

Although Robert had made sure English was John's first language to avoid him being beaten at school for speaking Welsh, we know that John did speak some Welsh, as he went to chapel and understood the services. At the chapel, services would have been a lot more exciting than in the English church where most of the service was the same words repeated every time. Through the nineteenth century there had been a series of revivals in Wales where charismatic nonconformist preachers spoke very passionately and converted a lot of people to Christianity.

Both John and Nye Bevan would later go on to use the charismatic Welsh chapel speaking techniques. The most important was *hwyl*, pronounced 'hoy-ull', which these days in modern Welsh means 'fun', but in the charismatic context means 'spirit' or 'a surge of intense emotion'.

By speaking on topics that they and listeners were passionate about, charismatic preachers could use the technique of *hwyl* to whip people up into a fervour of emotion and convert them to their cause. The tradition was to develop an argument, building up a speech a sentence at a time, each one a key part of the argument and relying on the sentence before, to make a final point. While circling round the topic, coming closer and closer, the speaker would also raise the emotional pitch by gradually speaking more loudly, passionately and emotionally. This meant that the whole speech had to be listened to: it could not be edited into soundbites when television came in, which is something that certainly held back Bevan, according to his biographer.[18] John, however, having the benefit of an English secondary education, was able to switch from *hwyl* into a more modern style when required, stating a summary of a point at the start of each paragraph and then expanding on it so that his points could be more easily noted and edited by others.

First public speaking to promote friendly societies

On 8 March 1892, it was John's turn to present at the Mutual Improvement Society, 'an excellent paper on "Friendly Societies".'

In the same newspaper column, there is also an advert for army service with 'great prospects of promotion' being offered to eligible young men in the Montgomeryshire Militia 4th Battalion, the South Wales Borderers. This was just after the first Boer War and the second Boer War would take place seven years later. These two wars would highlight the effects of semi-starvation in the workhouses since the 1830s on the health of young men: many were too weak and sickly to fight effectively. While the Conservative leaders at the time did not care too much for the health of poor people, in this case it affected the war – a key topic of interest, as losing a war would mean they might lose their lands. This influenced the sea change in public opinion which led to social reforms including the first old age pensions, national insurance and national health insurance.

It was in August 1892 that John became assistant clerk to the Forden Union workhouse, supporting his employer Sidney Pryce. John's first meeting is recorded in the local newspaper, with his father Robert also present as the relieving officer. The first item on the agenda was statistics, appropriately enough as this was what John went on to spend his career working on. Was this something that grew on him over time?

Amounts paid in out-relief during the past fortnight:—
Mr Robert Tomley, Montgomery, £14 4s 8d to 77 recipients;
Mr J. Fortune, Welshpool, £11 1s 7d to 61; Mr J. Oliver, Worthen,

£10 10s 8d to 76; non-resident poor, 8s to 2: total, £36 4s 11d to 220; against £36 0s 10d to 263, in the corresponding period of last year. Vagrants relieved during the fortnight, 134, as against 97; number in the house, 96, against 101. Amount of treasurer's balance due to the Union, £348 2s 1d.

The same report shows the board's compassion:

Col. Twyford said that while visiting the [Forden Workhouse] several inmates had asked him whether they could have a little more milk with their food, with their tea for instance in the morning, and also instead of soup one or two nights in the week. He understood that there was plenty of milk in the house – something more than was required – and under these circumstances he thought the request of the inmates ought to be acceded to. – The Master was instructed to supply milk to all who wished it.[19]

By April 1894, a report of another Forden board of guardians meeting shows what local people wanting to reform the workhouses were up against, even if they had an MP in the family in the case of Sir Pryce Pryce-Jones's son, who was on the board. An inspector 'was much surprised that the inmates were given boiled meat all year round, and he did not see why the meat could not be served in different forms', but the master of the workhouse and the chairman of the board were clearly resistant to change.[20] John would have learned from this a lot about the politics involved when dealing with committees. As assistant clerk he had likely written the minutes and been told by the chair to take out a suggestion from Pryce-Jones to improve the health of people in the workhouse so that it was buried and forgotten.

Sidney's wedding

In September 1892, John's boss Sidney Pryce's wedding to Mary Medlicott Newill was reported in the paper. John gave the happy couple a biscuit box and the Forden workhouse gave them an inkstand. It sounds a very fashionable affair, with the bridesmaids wearing Liberty silk dresses, quite fitting for Sidney, who liked to make a splash.

This was probably quite different to John's own tastes, which were much more modest. As a wedding guest, I wonder what he made of it all.

There were a number of well-to-do guests, including David Davies' wife (grandmother to the David Davies who John would later work with) and the bride's family on the Medlicott side, a local gentry family related very distantly to Winston Churchill and Princess Diana, although our branch didn't get the land or money. In stark contrast, the Newill side came from much humbler beginnings. Mary's father was Henry Starr Newill, whose mother, Elizabeth Starr, had had to run a post office to make ends meet after her husband died when Henry was four. Mary's cousin Clara, a bridesmaid, was related to author Geraint Goodwin's father.[21]

This is also how the solicitor's firm at Bishop's Castle, run by Henry Starr Newill, came into the Pryce, Tomley and Pryce firm, when Henry later passed it on to his son-in-law Sidney. This is the firm that my mum later took over and renamed Snows. After my mum's time, it later became Medlicott Snows, which is a satisfying coincidence considering that the original Mr Newill was married to a Medlicott.

Sidney and Mary went on their honeymoon in the North of England. While they were away, there was a fire near the Forden Workhouse. A fire broke out at the Gaer farm next door, and the 'fire queens' belonging to the workhouse were used to help tackle it. The next year, 1893, John joined the new Montgomery Fire Brigade set up by the council as a volunteer fireman, a role he would play for ten years, although they had no budget for equipment and had to collect donations.

The same year, John helped restart Montgomery Football Club, which he later became captain of, and won first prize in a bicycle race. He kept up with his cricket too, scoring second highest of the match while playing for nearby Chirbury. But then disaster struck. 'The wicket was a very bumpy one, and Copson's hands were badly battered, but poor Tomley had an awful crack on the head and it is a good thing for him that he has quite his share of brains, for some of them must have been badly disturbed by the severe blow. The next ball bowled him and no wonder.'[22]

July went from bad to worse. John's reflexes may have been affected by his bump on the head, as he was then involved in a cart accident when being given a lift by his friend Robert Bunner. The Montgomery County Times reported that 'Both occupants were thrown out, and [John] was dragged a considerable distance, his macintosh having caught in part of the vehicle, and the wheel passed over his shoulder... It is most miraculous that both gentlemen escaped without having any bones broken.'[23]

John must have recovered quite quickly as he is mentioned as being on the team at the cricket match a week later. He continued on the cricket team and was described the next year as 'the most promising young player in the team'.[24] Over the next fourteen years, John would keep playing: by August 1906, his team managed a crushing defeat of the much larger Newtown team, with John now doing most of the bowling. John was presented with a cup for his excellent bowling that season, and soon took over from Sidney as captain of the team.

John also remained firm friends with Robert Bunner, who would later be the best man at John's wedding. Today, the Bunners still own the hardware shop next door to John's old solicitors office on Arthur Street, and remained friends of the family ever since.

John Lloyd, known to our family as 'Uncle John' because he later acted as guardian to my father and his brothers after their own parents had died, was a later Mayor of Montgomery and a historian, as well as a national LGBTQ icon. Forty years later, he recorded some memories of Robert Bunner from local Montgomery resident Hannah Jones. What is clear from these memories is that Rob was a great choice of friend for John Tomley – someone with strong views who John could sharpen his debating skills with.[25]

Oddfellows secretary

August 1893 brought better news for John. He stood for his first Oddfellows appointment, as secretary of his local branch in Montgomery, and won the election by 48 votes to 16. At 19, John was now the youngest Oddfellows branch secretary in the country.[26]

Twenty-year-old John then gave a detailed talk on friendly societies at Berriew Mutual Improvement Society in the Assembly Rooms at Efel Fach, which was reported in several local newspapers. This was his first public speech on the subject of the Five Giants, which would occupy the rest of his career. It is clear that the young John had learned well and had absorbed a great deal of the detailed political arguments of the time.

First John introduced the history of friendly societies. Next he moved on to a brand new idea – old-age pensions, which didn't exist in those days. At the Montgomery Oddfellows branch, John was hoping to start a pension scheme for the very first time, using their surplus investments, to give local older people a weekly pension of 5 shillings or more. 'Dealing with the question of old-age pensions, he said that it was within comparatively recent years that this had been made a national question and the light of the most brilliant stars in the political firmament had been showered on it with more or less illuminating power.' A Royal Commission had been set up to report on the 'aged poor' and what could be done. Funding was a key issue – most branches of friendly societies had not done as well as Montgomery so government funding was required to cover people who were already of pension age. Other people currently working would have the opportunity to contribute to pensions so that it was 'the interest on a judicious investment and not as a gratuity doled out to a cringing pauper'.

The grand master of the Oddfellows, their national leader, was very keen to keep old-age pensions as something administered by friendly societies, even if a government old-age pension fund were to be formed. Here we see the friendly society bosses protecting their turf from the government, an issue which would become less of a problem later once a Liberal government was in power from 1906 onwards.[27]

According to the *Wrexham Advertiser*, John said that through friendly societies 'men and women, too, could secure the payment of a pension on reaching the age of sixty-five, instead of merely trusting to their sick pay. Therefore, in the course of another generation or two the only persons that would have to be provided for would be those who had been culpably negligent, or who had been the victims of some cruel misfortune. It seemed a very hard thing to send to the workhouse an honest, hard-working man, who had lived respectably all his life, and it seemed hard to give him the very bare pittance of outdoor relief.'[28]

The *Oddfellows Magazine* explains a useful connection John had made here with the chair of the debate, Mr. A.C. Humphreys-Owen, barrister-at-law, chairman of the county council and quarter sessions. He was a member of the government's Royal Commission on the Aged Poor.[29]

Two years later, at the annual meeting of his lodge, John as secretary reported that it was in a very strong financial position with £21 saved up per member, and the actuary had said they had £3,000 more than they need to pay out for estimated future sick pay, which could be used for more benefits. John suggested investing the money and using its returns to pay old-age pensions. In those days, people simply worked until they dropped dead. If they were too ill to work, people relied on the support of their children, or were sent into the workhouse.

The same year, John's keenness to take on many voluntary roles suddenly had to be balanced with the reality of his law studies. He had to resign his post as cricket club secretary and treasurer as he no longer had time to do everything. Was John going to have enough time to study for and pass his legal exams, or was he still doing too much?

Montgomery Town Council

John's work at the council continued, assisting the clerk, Sidney Pryce. One of Sidney and John's roles was running parliamentary and local council elections, including making sure everyone eligible was informed there was an election and could vote, that the votes were kept secret and the counting of votes was accurate.

In July 1892, John got to play a part in an election for the first time, when he was the assistant officer helping count the votes for the parliamentary seat of Montgomery Boroughs (then a separate seat to Montgomeryshire), although John couldn't vote himself.[30] It is notable that there were only 303 voters on the register, in a town of over 1,000 people. Only property-owning men could vote and unsurprisingly they tended to vote for wealthier candidates like themselves. Local mail order inventor and tycoon Sir Pryce Pryce-Jones was returned as the Conservative MP. The Pryce-Jones family had gone dramatically up in the world after recently making their fortune, and had now become part of 'the elite'. This was a source of some jealousy and irritation to everyone else, who had to wait many years for a meritocracy to sweep them up the social ladder too.

In July 1895, another general election took place and Major Edward Pryce-Jones, son of Sir Pryce, took on his father's parliamentary seat. John presided over the voting at the Machynlleth polling station. The Conservative majority over the Liberals was reduced from 118 to 84 voters.

In September, the local paper reported that John had applied to become a voter, but was not allowed, probably because he did not own any property at this point. This is likely to be a key factor in his later support of the Liberals, who were pushing to extend the vote to all men. Yet John was assistant clerk at the council. To find out whether he was eligible to vote, he only needed to ask Sidney at their office. There was no need for John to go through the process of applying in order to find out. This makes me wonder whether it was a politically motivated act by John to deliberately apply and be turned down, in order to draw attention to the unfairness of the rules. If so, was this something his friends the suffragettes might have suggested to him?

As well as elections, John also needed to take responsibility for balancing the books, managing the council's public finances. In 1897, John started presenting the annual accounts to Montgomery Town Council and recommending the rates level needed to cover the budget for spending for the coming year. This was complex work because the budget needed was tricky to predict in advance – especially if some kind of emergency happened mid-year. John also helped to collect the rates.

Progress at the Oddfellows

In November 1898, John's suggestion as secretary to the Montgomery branch of the Oddfellows, that their surplus was used for old-age pensions, was successfully agreed as one of the options open to each member. This was John's first big policy win. Shortly afterwards, John was appointed to a new Oddfellows role, as public auditor for Montgomeryshire, the whole county, under the Friendly Societies Act. This was on the recommendation of the new MP, Colonel Edward Pryce-Jones, whose Royal Welsh Warehouse team often played John's Montgomery team at cricket.

In June 1900, John went to the Annual Moveable Conference of Oddfellows, their national conference, for the first time, attending on behalf of Montgomeryshire. The *Oddfellows Magazine* records that he spoke briefly at the conference, proposing better auditing standards. John's proposal was rejected, yet he gained valuable experience of debating at a national meeting. Back at his local branch in Montgomery, John reported on the conference proceedings and won a prize for recruiting the highest number of new members for their branch.

July 1901 was the diamond jubilee of the Oddfellows Lodge at Montgomery, with lunch and speeches held in a marquee at Lymore. The grand master of the Oddfellows, the national leader, visited, and Mr A.C. Humphreys-Owen, now a local MP, gave a particularly provocative speech about the disadvantages of state support with pensions. The government would have to check if their local branches were solvent, interfering with their work, and if people were helped with pensions then other people practising thrift should be helped too, and where would it stop? John was hosting so had to be polite to his face, yet was probably stirred to a greater determination to improve pensions by adding state support.[31]

End of the century

The last year of the nineteenth century was one of bereavement for both John and Sidney.

In March 1899, Sidney's nine-month-old son Geoffrey died. He was Sidney and Mary's third child, following Vaughan in 1894 and their daughter Noel in 1895.

John covered for Sidney as clerk at a meeting of Forden Rural District Council to help. In contrast to Montgomery Town Council's medical officer reports, those by the medical officer at Forden, C.P. Moreton, were much more comprehensive and John's eyes were opened to the power of statistics in health. At the March meeting, the medical officer gave statistics about deaths, showing that infant deaths under one year old in the area were 8.4 per cent, an improvement on the average over the past 18 years of 10.1 per cent, although Sidney and his wife had still been unlucky with their baby son. The medical officer had also investigated and isolated cases of scarlet fever and diphtheria. The sanitary inspector had visited 972 houses. The Talbot Inn in Berriew had improved its sanitation. The suspected well at the school in Berriew had improved and the water closets there been much improved. This might have been the reason that a new school was built in Berriew which opened fifteen years later – where I later went to primary school. Sadly, after all Dr Moreton's hard work, he died within a year, so sanitary standards slipped back again.

There was more to come. John's mother Esther died in September 1899, at the age of 57, after a long and painful illness. The floral tributes sent to her funeral included one from Edith Soley, John's future wife, who supported John at this difficult time for him.

January 1900 saw the start of a new century, but it was nothing like when we all partied in 1999. The second Boer War had started in South Africa and fundraising was going on to support the wives and families of men serving abroad. John attended a Send-Off Supper for the volunteers from Montgomery Cricket Club. As he was articled at the time to Sidney, he could not join the army himself. The Mutual Improvement Society debated the subject 'Is the war with the Transvaal justifiable?' with John on the affirmative side. John had also joined the local volunteer army corps. By January 1901, Queen Victoria died and her son, Edward VII, became king. The Victorian era was over and the Edwardian era had begun.

In 1901, there was good news at last for Sidney Pryce and his wife Mary. They had a healthy baby girl, my grandmother Sydney Mary. Sidney was so pleased that he called her after himself, giving her what to everyone sounded like a male name and perhaps causing Sydney to want to be a tomboy. He actually misspelt her name on her birth certificate as the male version. His own name had been misspelt on his christening certificate as the female version as well. Sydney loved hunting and shooting in later life. As a baby, however, she was fussed over by her parents, dressed up like a little doll, and put in a wicker hamper to have a photo which they used for their Christmas cards.

Pirate bride

John and Edith decided to get married in April 1902. John had just qualified as a solicitor, one of 17 of the 113 candidates to gain honours in his exams, after ten long years of training. John was now able to handle legal cases in his own right and began to do well for his clients in court. He was also able to become a partner in Sidney's law firm so now had the means to support a family. They later renamed the firm Pryce, Tomley & Pryce.

I imagine Sidney, a Conservative, may have been a little surprised by his younger partner John's Liberal and increasingly outspoken socialist views as his mission to support social welfare grew, not to mention John's then unfashionable pride in his Welsh heritage. Despite this, Sidney and John must have got on well as business partners because they worked together for the rest of their working lives.

After John's mother died, he and his father Robert needed a housekeeper. There were no labour-saving devices or ready meals in those days, so working men had to pay for someone to cook and clean for them. In close contact each day and grieving his wife, Robert had soon started a relationship with the housekeeper, Mary Ann Hotchkiss, and they quickly got married. This was awkward for John to now have a stepmother so soon after his mother's death. He was keen to fly the nest and get married as soon as possible.

John was 28 and Edith was 24. They knew each other well through going to chapel together their whole lives, and had also taken part in many youth activities together including music and drama performances. Edith still lived above the grocer's shop on the same street as John's office, so they saw each other in passing every day too. Edith had been particularly kind to John around the time of his mum's illness and death, and they became even closer. Finally, John proposed and she accepted.

Traditionally, weddings were not allowed in the Welsh chapels due to English laws, so had to take place in the Church of England parish church. By this time, some chapels were allowed to carry out weddings, but the local chapel may not have applied for a licence yet.

Edith 'looked charming in a pretty dress of white corded silk, trimmed with lace chiffon, and wore a wreath of orange blossoms'. John gave her a bouquet of white roses and lilies of the valley. The four bridesmaids included Grace Tipping, the local schoolmaster's daughter. Robert Bunner was John's best man.

As the happy couple left the church, confetti was thrown, the church bells were rung, and cannons were fired. This was before the days of health and safety! Fortunately, they all arrived safely at the reception at the Town Hall. Later that afternoon John and Edith left by train for Liverpool and then spent their honeymoon in Scotland.

As was typical, the presents were very practical. Compared to Sidney's long list of wedding presents, John's is even longer at two-thirds of a column in the newspaper, showing how popular he and his father Robert were. John's father gave a cheque, John's stepmother gave a tea service, Robert Bunner gave a walnut overmantel, Sidney Pryce gave a dessert service. As well as close family and friends, there were presents from many staff at Forden Workhouse, the council and local MP Colonel Pryce-Jones. The local police officer gave dessert spoons and a farmer gave a beef tongue – in those days a delicacy. The Oddfellows clubbed together to buy a walnut roll-top writing desk.[32]

At that time of John and Edith's wedding, Edith was young, healthy and beautiful. There was no suggestion of the genetic disease, Huntington's disease, that she would later develop and pass on down the family line, and which two of their three children would die from.

The history passed down the family is that the Soleys were descended from French pirates. My granny Jose, John's daughter-in-law, always maintained that it was true. Modern genealogy has revealed that this is a definite possibility. Many people from the countryside in mid Wales worked at sea, there were certainly privateers in the family – the more respectable version of pirates – and the name Soley has French origins.

Huntington's disease has been likened to a pirate curse, where the curse keeps on going through generations of a family – perhaps for seven generations. We've had four generations that we know of, so maybe the pirates were three generations back from that? Happily medical science has meant we haven't had to travel to some underwater cave over the other side of the world to undo the curse, and my daughter has been the first generation to benefit.

Soon after John and Edith's wedding, Edith became pregnant. Their first child, Esther, was born in February 1903, followed in July 1905 by Edith Doris, my mum's Aunt Doris. Despite two toddlers under her feet, Edith stayed involved with local community activities such as organizing teas with the mayor's wife, a useful addition to John's own networking efforts.

The 1911 census shows John Tomley, aged 37, with his wife Edith, aged 33, and children Esther, 8, Doris, 5, and my grandfather Edward as a new baby. We have a lovely black and white photo of Edith holding baby Edward which must have been taken that year. John was working as a solicitor and the family were living at 3 Alexandria Terrace in Montgomery, so had moved out from his parents' home.

By the time of the 1921 census, the family had moved to The Hollies on Kerry Road in Montgomery, which became their long-term home. The house had been built in the 1700s. John bought it from the suffragette Farmer sisters we met earlier. It was from his study at The Hollies that John carried out much of his work in laying the foundations for the NHS, using the desk given to him by the Oddfellows to celebrate his marriage. We still have a matching desk which was in my childhood home, and the other must have been sold at some point without anyone noticing the inscription. This desk went to America and my uncle was recently contacted by the person who now owns it, to ask if he was a relative of John Tomley. It was from that desk that John's great achievements would begin.

Chapter 2

'An Antidote to Pauperism'
1906–1911

Fired up by his involvement in growing local friendly society membership in his local area of Montgomeryshire, on 14 February 1906, 32-year-old John wrote a long and persuasive article extracted in a local newspaper, the *Border Counties Advertizer*, about fighting poverty: 'Pauperism and its Antidote in Montgomeryshire'. John set out his stall with characteristic eloquence:

> Here, in the quiet backwater, as it were, of Montgomeryshire, remote from the rushing tide of strenuous life, that thrusts weaker humanity to the wall in the great centres of industry, can be studied under normal conditions the causes that lead to pauperism and the tendencies that steer clear of its stigma. A familiar acquaintance from childhood with both of these great features of our national life – Friendly Society work and Poor Law administration – may make me near-sighted in attempting a summary of their contrasts, but it is probably this very experience that has prompted my friend the editor to invite me to grapple with the subject.

The article refers to the newly formed Labour Party. At the time it was not expected that the Labour Party would win many votes, so the party of reform still effectively remained the Liberals, which John supported. Montgomeryshire was a strongly Liberal constituency. The election which ran to 8 February 1906 resulted in a Liberal landslide majority against the Conservatives across the UK, including 26-year-old mining heir David Davies winning the Montgomeryshire seat. This meant that the Liberal Party were able to consider passing legislation to achieve social reform.

A week after the election, John wrote his article. It must have taken him several weeks at least to assemble the statistics by writing letters to relevant friendly society colleagues, so he must have planned it in advance before the election result was known. Appropriately for Valentine's Day, the theme was caring for others. The article was so popular it was reprinted as a separate leaflet priced at 1d. and the resulting letters attached, including praise from two MPs.

John was inspired to write the article after listening to a speech by Tom Mills, an Oddfellows leader who was campaigning for TB sanatorium treatment.

It is notable that everything suggested in the article was achieved in John's lifetime and to a large extent as a result of his efforts: the introduction of old-age pensions, universal unemployment support, universal healthcare.

Even the audit of friendly societies by a 'skilled official auditor' mentioned by the leader writer, came to pass. I was very surprised to read that John was an auditor. As an accountant in a family of solicitors, I had thought I was the only auditor in the family. I started my career auditing charities nearly a century later in 2001, with clients including a friendly society.

Women had started to be allowed to join the Oddfellows as members in their own right the previous year, so society was moving forward.[1] As the majority of people in poverty were women, the Oddfellows now represented a real option for solving poverty for everyone.

John had also started to be nominated for the Oddfellows' powerful national body, the Investigation Committee, in 1903, although it was still another few years yet before he would finally manage to get elected.[2] John could see how people like him could perhaps start to grasp the levers of power to change things for the better for everyone.

The reference to 'pauperism' may seem to be rather insulting language to us. Yet this was the official legal language of the day, over a century ago, for people without any money at all. The efforts of John Tomley and others changed the language that we use about people on lower incomes. Within a few years after this article was published, the introduction of old-age pensions turned things around for a large percentage of the paupers, who had been mainly older people, and now enjoyed a minimum income in retirement. The foundation of the welfare state effectively eradicated pauperism for everyone else – people of working age and children – because everyone was now entitled to a guaranteed minimum income, food and a roof over their head.

Pauperism and Its Antidote in Montgomeryshire

'PAUPERISM AND ITS ANTIDOTE IN MONTGOMERYSHIRE
A STATISTICAL ARTICLE

By J. E. Tomley, Assistant Clerk to the Forden Union and Public Auditor of Friendly Societies

The newspaper's introduction to John's article observed:

> There is a general expectation that for good or evil the new Parliament will be distinguished above all its predecessors for its attempts to improve the condition of the people... Everything, therefore, points to what we may call a parliament of social legislation...
>
> For this reason we value very highly papers like Mr Tomley's, [which] have the greatest merit in being written in that lucid and interesting way which helps to tempt the public to read what they would otherwise pass by as too hard and dry.

The paper then summarized the extent of funds held by the friendly societies, along with cooperative and building societies: across 18 million members in total, there was around £400 million 'standing to the credit of the working classes'. It added:

> So much for thrift and savings. On the other hand, in the year ending March last 816,216 persons were in receipt of poor relief in England and Wales at a cost of £6,366,304.

Extracts from John's own analysis followed, 'showing the effect of Friendly Societies in reducing pauperism', backing his case up with statistics at every point. John wrote, for example:

> A striking fact is elicited by taking an imaginary line drawn from Plynlymon to Llanfyllin, dividing the county into two portions. To the north and west of this line less than 8 per cent of the population belong to friendly societies, and out-relief costs 4s per head; to the south and east over 15 per cent are members of friendly societies, and the cost of out-relief is only 2s 2d per head. Another telling argument in favour of membership of friendly societies as a preventative of pauperism is realized when we find that only eighteen persons out of the 1,993 who received relief in the county last year belonged to any friendly society.

John observed that locally, in the parishes around the Forden Union workhouse where he and his father had worked hard to increase friendly society membership, 'only £827 was administered in out-relief in the past twelve months, while no less than £2,765 was paid out in benefits by the friendly societies in the same parishes. The proportion is reversed for the remainder of the county...' In a total local population around Montgomery of around 4,500, there were 'only thirteen male paupers, whose average age is over 75, and none of them belong to a benefit club'.

The newspaper reporter reminded readers that 'the work of the friendly societies in lessening the burden of poor relief entitles them to the support of those who benefit from reduced rates' – i.e. friendly societies should be given local government funding – and continues:

> Mr Tomley adds another cogent reason why tradesmen should become members and urge those in their employ to do the same, and it is this: that in times of sickness it is often the club money which enables the tradesmen's customers to pay their debts.

The piece concluded with suggesting that friendly societies' accounts should be examined by a 'skilled professional auditor': 'The societies play so large and important a part in the affairs of the nation that the soundness of their finances is a matter of national concern.'[3]

John's full article provided several statistical tables and commentary on them, clearly showing that the friendly societies in their current form, providing affordable and reliable health insurance and unemployment insurance for low-paid workers, were a key part of the solution to eradicate the depredations of the Five Giants.

John's figures also showed the business case for friendly society membership. By helping people through times of sickness and unemployment from their own savings, there was less reliance on Poor Law relief paid by the local ratepayers. His powerful argument continued:

> The poor are always with us, and the ever-present problem of the aged poor, though dissected by Royal Commissions and subjected to minor surgical treatment by countless individuals, seems far from being solved; yet, indeed, it deserves the attention of the State far more than most of the questions that have excited the country in recent years.

John also looked at the thorny question of state aid, on which 'the friendly societies are somewhat divided', arguing that the societies needed to unite with a common purpose, declining 'to initiate any person who was not prepared to insure for sick benefit up to sixty years of age, and for superannuation benefit afterwards':

> When working men had by their thrift secured a superannuation after sixty years of age, the State ought to pay them an equal amount. By this means the rates would be relieved and the old-age pension problem solved.

Published in the booklet with the reprinted article were many letters of support received by John from MPs and others.

William Charles Bridgeman, the new Conservative MP for Oswestry, said John's article 'affords much ground for reflection' and realized the wider potential: 'If similar statistics could be compiled for other counties it would be valuable.' John David Rees, the new Liberal MP for Montgomery Boroughs, said that John had performed 'a great public service'. And Colonel Edward Pryce-Jones, who had just lost that seat, also wrote in support of John's 'able, clear and statistical paper'.

Many Oddfellows district leaders responded, too. Mr H. Hughes, secretary of the Shrewsbury District of Oddfellows, said: 'What a revelation! You have dealt with the matter in so lucid and masterly a manner that the article will be an eye-opener to most thinking people.' It seems one of the other district leaders passed the article on to Mr E.F. Hind, past national grand master of the Oddfellows, who responded from Manchester: 'Your article is most interesting and valuable... I trust something practical will result from your effort, for which many will thank you.'[4]

John's article rightly suggested friendly society membership could solve pauperism, yet there was still the issue that not every working man was included because some people chose not to join. Whether people joined or not made no difference to their chance of needing healthcare, so there would still be people with no healthcare.

Friendly societies only provided a doctor's appointment and, in most cases, did not stretch to hospital treatment. The rest of the family were also not covered, so in the case of contagious illnesses such as TB, other family members could remain ill and continue to spread the disease, including reinfecting the working man of the household.

One of the biggest issues with friendly societies was the risk, mentioned in John's article, of people joining a friendly society which was unable to pay for the health and other benefits due, and therefore went bust. This was particularly likely in hard-pressed areas with high unemployment, or areas with a large population of older people where young people had moved to work in England. A government-backed state scheme, covering the whole of the UK would mean that areas with high unemployment could be subsidized by areas which were doing better.

Shortly after his election in February 1906, John announced to the Montgomery branch of the Oddfellows that David Davies MP, had expressed his intention of joining them, as had John David Rees MP. The next year, Davies would offer a prize in the paper to the people recruiting the most new members for their friendly society branches in Montgomeryshire. He was one of the youngest MPs, at just 26 years old.

This is the first time John and David are recorded as working together. They became firm friends and would spend the rest of their careers as close colleagues.

John quickly involved David in political campaigning to eradicate pauperism, and fundraising for health and welfare; for example, raising money to build the new Montgomeryshire Infirmary hospital at Newtown.

National recognition

In April, John's article on 'Pauperism and its Antidote' started to get picked up in the national press. *The Manchester Guardian* (renamed *The Guardian* in 1959) reported:

> Bro. J. E. Tomley, secretary of the 'Loyal Ark of Friendship' Lodge, Montgomery, of the Manchester Unity of Oddfellows, has contributed an able and informative article to the press on 'Pauperism and its antidote,' in which he shows the great social work which friendly societies are doing, and their beneficent influence in cultivating habits of independence and in reducing pauperism. According to the 'Oddfellows' Magazine,' carefully compiled statistics are given as to the amount paid in sickness benefits by the friendly societies. The article has aroused widespread interest in the district in which it was published, and it should prove helpful to the friendly societies and to the community.' [5]

May 1906 saw John appear in the *Guardian* again, continuing his campaigning for old-age pensions and state support. The article explained the question 'is of such vital importance to friendly societies generally, that, in response to a request made to us from several quarters we have decided to publish a more extended report of the able and interesting address of Bro. J. E. Tomley, solicitor, of Montgomery, by whom the subject was introduced.'

John went on to explain that a proposal for an endowment fund to provide old-age pensions had come from the Montgomery district. The friendly societies in the UK did not receive any state aid. In contrast, in other countries, such as Germany, Denmark, Belgium, France and New Zealand, successful state-aided old-age pension schemes had been set up. These had successfully reduced the number of older people living in poverty. The newspaper continued:

> He was afraid that old-age pensions in this country were a political Will-o'-th'-wisp, and that the cost to the State, which they had been estimated to amount to sixteen millions per annum by the year 1921, made it appear prohibitive to successive Chancellors of the Exchequer.
>
> As was stated in our report of the Conference, Bro. Tomley's speech created a most favourable impression upon the delegates, and there was a general consensus of opinion in favour of the establishment of a Unity Endowment Fund on the lines suggested.[6]

Shortly afterwards, at the Oddfellows' Annual Moveable Conference in Barrow, John spoke five times in the national debate on this subject.[7]

Empty of paupers?

In June 1907, John organized the Montgomery District Oddfellows' diamond jubilee – marking sixty years of the district. Grand Master Bro. Dempsey, the national leader of the Oddfellows, came to Montgomery. John said that through the work of the friendly societies, the workhouses will soon be empty of paupers.

A few months later, John explained to the Forden Workhouse board of guardians that the number of people in their casual ward had halved compared to last year. He also showed the board the first national statistics for Wales which had been produced for workhouses, showing that Forden had the cheapest cost per head of population, partly due to having an amalgamated service covering a relatively large area. John no doubt took all this in when later recommending a national approach as being more effective for delivering health services.

A few years earlier, in 1904, John's father Robert had been appointed to the assessment committee of the Forden board of guardians, in the place of the late Mr E.R. James, who had been mayor of Montgomery. It seemed like a social revolution was starting: Robert, who had many years' experience of running the workhouse, was appointed instead of the usual rich property owners who had sat on these boards up to now.

In September 1908, John became provincial grand master of the Montgomery District of Oddfellows, responsible for the whole county. This was a remarkable achievement for a 34-year-old. John continued his campaigning on old-age pensions, addressing the Three Counties annual conference on this topic, and urging them not to object to state pensions.

Clerk to the county pensions committee

The Old-Age Pensions Act was passed by the Liberal government in 1908, after much campaigning by John and others. The first pensions were now available for all older people across the UK. The rate was set low, the equivalent to £23 per week today, to encourage people to keep making their own pensions savings too.

Everyone who wanted a pension had to apply to a local pension committee starting in October 1908, and the pensions started from 1 January 1909. John was appointed as clerk to the Pensions Committee of Montgomeryshire County Council, managing all the pensions applications and payments for the county.

This first Pensions Act offered state pensions for men and women who were over 70, whose annual income was below £31 10s., and who had lived in the UK at least 20 years. There were a lot of holes in the act, as John acknowledged when he spoke publicly about it: starting at 65 would have been better, as many people got too ill to work from this age, and benefits from friendly societies counted against the means test. John suggested these issues could be ironed out when the law was next updated in future. If the UK was anything like other countries, after the initial pilot, the scheme would probably be rolled out further to cover more people. John said that the friendly societies 'must not fight against what the Government did for the benefit if the working people, but should try and get all the advantages possible for their members, and remove the disabilities under which they at present suffered.'[8]

By December 1908, the local paper reported 'Old-age pensions in Montgomeryshire – great number of claims'. Applications for the new pensions had flown in thick and fast to John, before the 1 January 1909 start date for the new scheme.[9] It was John's job as clerk to present the pensions applications to the committees deciding the claims for each local area in the county of Montgomeryshire, and recommend whether or not the pension should be given, which the committee would then discuss and confirm. Once the scheme had bedded in, it supported two-thirds of people over 70 in the county.

In April 1909, John spoke at the Three Counties Conference of the Oddfellows at Port Sunlight near Liverpool, calming fears about Chancellor of the Exchequer David Lloyd George's plans for the introduction of state pensions. Lloyd George – who of course had deep Welsh roots himself and was brought up speaking Welsh – had recently been to Germany and had been impressed by their compulsory state national insurance scheme which covered everyone. One of the Oddfellows directors warned that they, 'as directors of the Manchester Unity, had thought it their bounden duty to oppose compulsory national State insurance, and they issued a supplementary resolution to the various districts asking them to discuss the question, which, if passed into law, would sound the death knell of Friendly Societies.'

In the same issue of Oddfellows Magazine, it was reported John said that:

> The directors had become rather hysterical over the business. So far as he could see there was no definite proposal before the country, and what they had to consider were Mr. Lloyd George's impressions of Germany. The only thing which stood before the British public was the fact that a Royal Commission was to be appointed to deal with the working of Friendly Societies. They, as members of the Manchester Unity, would welcome such a commission, because they were bound to come out top in the end. [10]

In April 1910, John and Edith's third child was born, Edward George Soley Tomley. He was a much-longed-for son for John who could take over the family solicitors firm. It was therefore worth John building up the firm for Edward. The next month, John was at the Oddfellows' Annual Moveable Conference in Southampton. By this time he had become a member of his first UK-wide committee, the Oddfellows' Investigation Committee, which was responsible for issuing national hardship grants, governance and audit.

The highlight of the conference was the Oddfellows Centenary Banquet, chaired by the Prince of Wales, soon to become King George V. Yet on 17 May, the *Oddfellows Magazine* records John having been called home by telegram due to a family illness. His son Edward was just a few weeks old, and he or Edith may have been unwell. So did he manage to return in time to attend the banquet the next day? History does not record.[11]

Sanitary insanity

In the late 1800s and early 1900s, there were many sanitation issues across the whole of the UK, and these helped to cause illnesses such as TB, cholera and typhoid. With no running water or flushing toilets in homes, infection spread easily. In Montgomery for example, 'an open stream-cum-sewer ran from behind the houses on the north side of Broad Street', down the garden of the doctor's house, and through various streets including Arthur Street where John had his office.[12]

Dealing with sanitation and resulting health issues was complex. John's father Robert was the sanitary officer for Montgomery Town Council, a very part-time role with low pay and unpopular decisions to be made. For example, in 1903, there was a case of smallpox and the patient's next-door neighbour was told by Robert and the medical officer that he must isolate, and therefore could not work, so he complained a lot about the loss of earnings.

December 1906 saw an interesting meeting of Montgomery Town Council, who now seemed to be taking sanitation and diseases affected by living conditions, such as TB, a lot more seriously, a discussion John would have picked up on. All the issues which were later picked up in the 1930s TB inquiry were touched upon, including: the need for TB sanatoria where patients could have open-air treatment to recover; the risk factor of overcrowding in homes; councillors not liking to bring rich landlords such as J.M.E. Lloyd and Lord Powis to book about homes without proper toilets; part-time non-specialist sanitary inspectors; and other conflicts of interest such as the mayor owning the gas company and keeping the price of gas high. There was also a tendency for some councillors to put off important discussions to a future meeting, therefore preventing action being taken.

John's father Robert also resigned his role as the sanitary inspector. On his last meeting, he allowed himself a little smile. It was clearly requiring a lot of work and only paying him £5 per year, £650 in today's terms. He was also 72 years old, and had probably worked that long due to not having a pension, a factor that probably influenced John in his campaigning for pensions for everyone over 65. Robert had seven years of retirement and lived to age 79. For six years of that time, he enjoyed a small pension, thanks to John's campaigning.[13]

By 1907, the Forden board of guardians had also become more up to date on TB, asking about it at their board meeting, and were told that one person had consumption, on the men's sick ward. A member of the board asked whether they ought to be put in a separate ward. Another suggested, if the case was in the early stages, the patient might undergo an open-air sanatorium treatment, a new type of treatment which was becoming popular.

The Welsh National Memorial Association

In February 1910, David Davies had been re-elected as MP for Montgomeryshire. Fortunately for all the working people in the county, he had now declared his party allegiance as radical socialist, a new progressive section of the Liberal Party. There were a number of different parties and subsections of parties around at the time, as politics had been put into flux by the rise of the labour movement. One thing was quite clear, though: David wanted to make his mark and change the world for the better.

David's new allegiance quickly turned into a firm plan for him to make a philanthropic statement. He gave away £150,000 (£16.3 million in today's terms), a huge amount of his wealth, for the benefit of working people in need of healthcare. It also avoided having to wait for the government of the day to get round to doing something. As David's unpublished biography described it, 'Parliamentary methods were too slow and long-winded for his impetuous spirit.'[14]

In September 1910, David invited his friend John Tomley to the first meeting of what would later become the King Edward VII Welsh National Memorial Association. John had been expressing many radical socialist views over the past few years, so David knew he would have an enthusiastic supporter, as well as someone who knew about friendly society, local government and workhouse health administration. John was what is now known in the NHS and local government today as a 'boundary spanner', a person who can liaise between different parts of the system. They were both much younger than most of the men in power around them, the older Victorian generation. David was 30 and John was 36.

David and John saw themselves as kindred spirits, embracing modern ways, and supporters of emerging labour movement thinkers inspired by Marx, who had explained why the old capitalist order of bosses exploiting working people must go. They would have tossed about these new ideas together. While they were not going so far as to press for communism, they did think things should be made more equal, particularly for those who were most in need. They had also both been brought up as Calvinistic Methodists, taught from their earliest years to tithe and give money generously to help others, as well as being in touch with working Welsh people who sat with them in the Welsh chapel pews, in contrast to the more aloof churchgoers at the English church.

The death of King Edward VII, who had supported the idea of finding a cure for TB, gave David and John an opportunity to do something radical in that field, dressed up as a very unobjectionable Welsh memorial to the late king, as something the king would have wished for and had in fact suggested at one point. This was very politically savvy for the time, as it meant the new service could attract well-off donors who were more likely to have right-wing views.

David wanted a pre-meeting with the people he knew with the most sensible views, including John and local doctors, before they went to the more formal meeting with the Lord Mayor of Cardiff, John Chappell. This would mean that the proposals requested at the meeting with Chappell would be sensible and practical ones, which would be highly effective on the ground.

Scientifically, at this point, it was known how to diagnose TB and that it could be cured in some cases with a new approach called sanatorium treatment, if caught early, with the patient sleeping in a bed outdoors for a while. This was no doubt rather uncomfortable for the patient, yet a life-saving necessity at the time.

There was also a fashion for prevention being better than cure, and cheaper too, in all areas of life, from fire prevention to the prevention of cruelty to children. It was but a small logical step to extend this to the idea of prevention in health. Teaching people about the factors that led to TB, such as patients sharing beds and rooms with other members of the family, would help people avoid catching the disease in the first place. Of course, this assumed that they had a separate bed and room to sleep in.

After the success of his old-age pensions campaigning, John would have been enthused to have another topic of vital national importance to take on. He already knew about running health services at the workhouse and as

Oddfellows lodge secretary. With his legal mind and experience of committees, he also knew how to write strong and legally watertight resolutions, which would form the basis of a new charity as a legal entity, be approved by the Charity Commissioners in due course, and properly support the work on the ground. John was also motivated by the death of Tom Mills, the Oddfellows leader and the speaker who had inspired John to write 'Pauperism and its Antidote' in 1906. Tom had particularly been campaigning for TB sanatorium treatment at the time, and died of TB himself the year after. Faced with the loss of his mentor, John felt he must take steps to eradicate TB.

Although this was David's first time running healthcare services, he was already a governor of the new University of Wales at Aberystwyth, where he would later invite John and Nye Bevan to join him on the board. The university was a known hotspot for TB infections, due to students travelling from other areas. Across Wales, TB was the disease that caused the most deaths of young people such as students. This might be why David strongly agreed with John that it was time to tackle TB.[15]

At this time, I expect John probably thought it would take a few years and then things would move on significantly, as they had for old-age pensions. Little did he know that twenty-seven years later he would be calling for an inquiry into why TB rates in Wales had fallen less than in England, despite all their efforts.

The Welsh Gazette reported on that first pre-meeting ('consumption' refers of course to TB), listing the attendees including 'Mr J.E. Tomley, Montgomery, (representing the friendly societies)':

> The meeting was convened by Mr David Davies, and consisted of those known to be interested in the scheme of the memorial which, roughly, aims at three things – (1) education by means of lectures, demonstration, etc., in regard to consumption; (2) the provision of dispensaries and trained nurses for certain areas; (3) the provision of a sanitorium or sanitoria. The estimated cost is put at £250,000 to £300,000...
>
> Mr Davies explained that the conference was in no sense hostile to the conference to be called by the Lord Mayor of Cardiff [the next and more formal meeting to set up the scheme], but was held to prepare the ground and to facilitate matters at the conference. The Lord Mayor, he said, had asked for suggestions as to the form the national memorial should take, and the conference of that day made certain proposals and formulated a plan of campaign.

At the end of the meeting, David 'was deputed to see the Lord Mayor' and submit their proposals to him.[16]

Around this time, a new phrase was entering the health debate too. Dr Benjamin Moore, a doctor from Liverpool who founded the State Medical Association, suggested a 'National Health Service' in his 1910 book *The Dawn of the Health Age*.[17] John knew that specialist services like TB were more effective organized on a higher level than counties – perfect for a national health service pilot.

Another article about the first WNMA meeting makes clear that their idea from the outset was to set up the first ever national health service, covering the whole of Wales, including prevention and acute care, and focusing on TB. David Davies asked the group to pledge itself 'to do everything in its power to ensure the success of the memorial, the ultimate object is to stamp out tuberculosis in Wales'. A particular feature of the work would be the provision of sanatoria. A general committee would be appointed, including 'the Lord Mayor of Cardiff, the Lord Lieutenant of each county, the County Medical Officer of Health, together with two persons selected by each County Council in Wales and Monmouthshire'.

This second article was accompanied by '10 facts about tuberculosis', such as there were at least 40,000 deaths from it every year in England and Wales, costing the government £8 million, and that 200,000 suffered with the effects of the disease even if they survived it. But solutions were available: 'Sanatorium treatment, combined with the use of tuberculin properly given has greatly diminished the terrors of consumption, and increased the probability of cure.'[18]

I went to the National Library of Wales to look at the Welsh National Memorial Association (WNMA) papers. It was thought that these were buried on the site of the main WNMA building in Cardiff, when the NHS was formed in 1948. Tragically, David Davies had died in 1944, at age 64, four years before his and John's dream of a comprehensive national health service for everyone was realized.

When I held the papers in my hands, including the minute book recording that first meeting in Shrewsbury, I could smell the history of a century of work. Despite suggestions that the papers had been buried underground, I was glad John had decided to give them to the National Library of Wales instead, or the smell might have been even more historic. The minute book was just an ordinary office stationery book, like many of that time. It contained only one meeting, and was then blank. After that, the local committees of the WNMA had been set up.

As an accountant, I had held quite a few old books like this before. Yet none were like this one, which contained the very start of our first ever national health service. It was at once fantastically radical and uncannily prosaic. This how the world is nearly always changed: through administrative meetings and minute books. 'The flat ephemeral pamphlet and the boring meeting,' as W.H. Auden would later describe it.[19] Radical administration.

National Insurance Act 1911

Throughout 1910, the Oddfellows and other friendly societies had been discussing the new National Health Insurance Bill proposed by Lloyd George and the Liberals, including David Davies.

An Oddfellows meeting at Glasgow heard about the prospect of state national insurance, which the chair, Bro. D.H. MacDonald of Brandon Works, disagreed with: 'If this bill should be passed into law, he was sure it would put a premium on the vagabond, the thriftless, and the wastrel.' John bravely faced him down and explained clearly how the changes would benefit working people: 'If they did have a compulsory system by which everyone must contribute, it would be better than having wives and families half-starved during the illness of the husband.'[20]

The following year, in June 1911, John attended the Oddfellows Annual Moveable Conference, as usual, this time at Brighton. The grand master spoke strongly against state control of the friendly societies and the new National Insurance Bill which meant the Oddfellows would have to become an approved society. John proposed a motion which was unanimously resolved, that an invitation be given to the chancellor of the exchequer, Lloyd George, the Welsh Wizard, to attend one of the meetings during the conference week for the exchange of views on the bill. It was far sighted of John to be the one to make the suggestion, as this would also imply that John himself would go to the meeting with the chancellor, one of the most powerful politicians in the country.

Later in the conference, John spoke again in support of the new National Insurance Bill: he

> was delighted to have the opportunity, coming from the country from which the Chancellor hailed, of saying a word on behalf of this great measure. He did not share the pessimistic view which had been expressed in some quarters. He preferred

to believe that the object of the Chancellor was the good of the community rather than to offer up, as a sacrificial beast, the interests of the great friendly and provident societies. He considered Mr. Lloyd George was doing the very best thing that he and his Government could do to inculcate the living throb of their work into this great State scheme...

Would not the advantages of the scheme outweigh the small disadvantages that the scheme would impose? For that reason, it would be one of the greatest things that had ever happened. The brother from Aylesbury had given away the secret of a good deal of the opposition to this Bill when he said, 'We have made provision for ourselves.' Was that the principle of the Manchester Unity? Were they going to play the part of the Levite or of the Good Samaritan, and bear one another's burdens? (Cheers.)' [21]

In October 1911, John organized a meeting of all local friendly societies in the county of Montgomeryshire, at Welshpool. This was an opportunity for friendly societies working at the grassroots to input issues about the National Insurance Bill to David Davies, who was good friends with Lloyd George, and for David to influence Past Grand Master Bourne, a national leader of the Oddfellows, to help his members accept the bill. The Oddfellows were particularly concerned that private industrial insurance companies were going to be allowed to administer the state scheme, milking a profit from it, unlike the friendly societies which were not for profit. John also explained that 'the infliction of the three days' period during which sick pay would not be paid would be a serious injustice... to the members and their families, who would have to go without wages or sick pay for that time when necessaries were most needed.'

David Davies said:

they were told at the beginning that the principle of the Bill was that it should assist the voluntary societies. He thought that principle should not be lost sight of... As to the non-payment during the first three days of sickness, he confessed that it was very difficult matter. When the Bill was under consideration in the House of Commons every day some addition was urged which would increase the cost, and they were always told that if they were insisted on the Bill must be dropped. But after hearing the speeches that night he certainly thought there was a very strong case for reconsidering the question as to the three days. (Applause.) Then in regard to the collecting insurance companies, he certainly thought they should not be assisted out of the Government funds when they were carrying on a trade or business for profit, and he did not see why they should come within the scope of the Bill. (Loud cheers.)[22]

By December 1911 the opportunity to debate was over and the National Insurance Act 1911 was passed by Parliament. Now, for the first time, people working in particular industries would be protected from sickness and disablement, receiving medical treatment and sick pay.

Chapter 3

'Enough to Keep Body and Soul Alive'
1912–1922

The following year, in February 1912, John started delivering lectures on the new National Insurance Act 1911 at venues across Wales, on behalf of the National Health Insurance Commission (Wales). This was the precursor to the Ministry of Health, so this was John's first position working directly for national government.

John's role was to explain the new National Insurance Act rules to everyone in a local area, from workers paying National Insurance for the first time, to local approved societies administering the scheme, to doctors, employers and local politicians. The local approved societies would arrange a meeting for their members and invite one of the official lecturers from a list of forty-one across the UK. Seven of these lecturers were Oddfellows, and thirteen were based in Wales. John and the other lecturers had been on a course arranged by the Insurance Commissioners, the government's civil servants who led the new National Insurance schemes and were responsible for making all high-level decisions.[1]

Part I of the Act, health insurance, provided some workers with compulsory health insurance for the first time, providing people with medical treatment and sick pay. All workers who earned £160 per year were covered if they worked in particular industries. The worker gave 4 pence per week to the scheme, the employer paid 3 pence and the government paid 2 pence through general taxation. Lloyd George called it 'Ninepence for Fourpence'.

The campaign by John and David Davies to keep the profiteering cowboys out of health insurance provision had worked. Private insurers' high administrative fees could take up to half the money available for sickness benefits. Approved societies were mutual societies which were owned by the workers themselves, and partly volunteer run, keeping costs low for everyone in their time of need.

Separately to the health insurance aspects John was lecturing on, there was also another part of the National Insurance Act. Part II of the

Act provided compulsory unemployment insurance for a smaller number of workers, those in industries more prone to unemployment. The unemployment insurance was provided separately and not through the friendly societies. Unemployed workers could collect their unemployment benefit from a local labour exchange, where they would be referred to new jobs during their visit.

The friendly societies were previously the main bodies administering unemployment insurance, so the fact that they had been excluded by the government from managing this part of the new scheme was a bone of contention. John, on behalf of the Oddfellows, persuaded David Davies to spend some time lobbying for friendly societies to be allowed to manage unemployment insurance. This campaign did progress and friendly societies were eventually offered the option to manage this part of the scheme. However, after confidential talks with the Oddfellows' board and others, it was decided not to progress with the scheme and to let the government continue to manage it. John and David probably felt very frustrated at the time, after all the effort they had put in with lobbying. Yet this later turned out to be a very wise decision. By the 1930s, the entire unemployment insurance scheme for the whole country had gone bust, as unemployment soared in the Great Depression and claims outweighed people's previous contributions.

Local health commissioner

In May 1912 John started a permanent new role, leading on administering the new National Health Insurance across Montgomeryshire, working for the county council. John had now become a local health commissioner. This is a similar role to the NHS's clinical commissioning groups (CCGs), which have recently changed their name to integrated care boards (ICBs), for each local area today. John was now responsible for organising how money was spent on health locally. It was his job to make sure people now covered by National Health Insurance got value for money when it came to all health services, including panel doctors (GPs) and hospital services. This meant John had a lot of power to improve health services – in fact, that is still one of the main purposes of the commissioners' role today. As clerk, John was the lead member of staff, what today would be called the chief executive.

At the meeting which appointed John, the chair, Mr E. Jones, said that John 'had special fitness for the post. He had made the work of benefit societies a life study, and in administering the Act he would be on familiar ground. He had known Mr. Tomley well in other spheres of public work, and he had such a high opinion of his capacities that he felt sure he would discharge the duties to the entire satisfaction of everyone.' The motion was carried unanimously.[2]

The WNMA takes off

Meanwhile in February 1912, David and John's new WNMA national TB service was starting off well, with a medical director appointed for the 'Welsh Consumption Crusade', Dr Marcus Paterson from Frimley, regarded as one of the foremost authorities on the subject in the UK. The WMNA was also potentially going to get a big chunk of its revenue funding from the new National Insurance Act health funding, supported by the chancellor of the exchequer. Yet the head of the Local Government Board, Mr John Burns, opposed this. In the end, the funding continued to come through local authorities. As we shall see, letting local authorities have a stranglehold on funding caused serious issues for the WNMA further down the line, which eventually led to the formation of the NHS.[3]

David Davies' unpublished biography explains more about the work of the WNMA at this time. David's relationship with Lloyd George had had a rocky start, with David sometimes being ahead of Lloyd George in his thinking, and Lloyd George warning people in Wales to beware of 'worshipping the Golden Calf' (meaning David). Yet now, everything was going smoothly.

> David... saw Lloyd George and explained the scheme to him, reminding him of three famous young Welsh poets who had died of the disease. This recalled to his mind the loss... of a friend of his own youth in his native village and he not only gave the scheme his full approval, but decided to make sanatorium benefit a feature of his [National Health Insurance] Bill...
>
> The [WNMA's] Royal Charter was secured by the beginning of July 1912 and on Saturday, July 27th, the first meeting of the Governors was held at Llandrindod Wells, with David, who had been unanimously elected President, in the Chair. In his opening address he was able to say with legitimate pride that Wales now had a National University, a National Museum, a National Library and a great National Health Institution.

He did not say – though he could truthfully have done so – that in the establishment of at least three of these bodies he himself had played a leading part...

The educational campaign had been pressed forward with great energy... the demand for the Association's literature had been excellent... For administrative purposes the Principality had been provisionally divided into thirteen districts, each of which would be in charge of a tuberculosis physician, with a tuberculosis institute and visiting stations, which would be of the simplest kind, all unnecessary expense being scrupulously avoided. These stations would be the local centres or clearing houses for detecting and dealing with cases in the first instance. From there patients would, where necessary, be sent to one of the Association's sanatoria, and it was the ultimate aim of the governing body to erect two of these, one for South and one for North Wales. Meanwhile, to meet the immediate demand, arrangements were being made to secure the use of various existing Hospitals, established for other purposes...

For the next two years the [WNMA] was driven on its course with unrelenting energy by its now formidable President. In order that the work might be carried on under his personal supervision he had established the head office at Newtown, and staff dreaded the days when... David would ride up... at 8.30 or 9.00 in the morning, issue enough orders to keep the office going for a fortnight and call again a few hours later... expecting to find every item of the programme carried out...

The amount of work needed to make the scheme effective was formidable. Tuberculosis physicians and nurses had to be appointed for the thirteen districts and their conditions of service arranged. Here the difficulty was increased by a quarrel between the British Medical Association and the Local Government Board as to their remuneration of doctors under the Health Insurance Act. Sanatorium committees had to be appointed to each district, and hospital and sanatorium beds acquired from existing institutions pending the erection and equipment of the Association's new sanatoria; visiting stations had to be provided in every town and rural area throughout Wales; the difficult but all important question of domiciliary treatment had to be worked out in conjunction with the doctors and the BMA. There was a long wrangle with the Treasury about the type of expenditure to which the government's proportionate grants should apply. Counties seceded from the scheme and deputations had to be sent to lure them back. Neighbourhoods in which it was proposed to establish sanatoria protested and had to be placated, and all the time the educational campaign had to be carried forward and the endowment fund built up.[4]

During this time, John, as the local health commissioner for Montgomeryshire, was on the decision-making committees for the WNMA. John would have often been called upon to help marry up David's wish to push things forward with the practicalities of running health services on the ground day-to-day, where John had many years' experience. The WNMA boasted right from the start of being fully supported by the county councils, and John led on providing this support in Montgomeryshire and persuading the other councils across the country to support and fund the WNMA too. John also acted as a critical friend, explaining to David when he was pushing things too hard, what practical steps needed to be taken, and how best to achieve these.

Off to see the Wizard?

So, after the National Health Insurance Act was bedded in, did this mean John's policy and campaigning work was finished? After all, the key things he and David Davies had fought for were now in place, run by national government for the first time: old-age pensions, health insurance and unemployment insurance. These had been unthinkable a decade before, yet had now all been achieved by their radical socialist movement in the Liberals. After several years of hard work, now John could surely rest on his laurels for a bit.

Yet, of course, things didn't work out like that. Despite successful lobbying on some issues like excluding the private health insurers from National Insurance, many other issues remained with the National Insurance Act. One of the biggest holes was that not all working people were covered, only certain trades and lower earners. Sickness and disability struck at random – they did not care whether you were an employed fisherman (covered) or a self-employed gardener (not covered). Some more specific issues, like the three days unpaid at the start of sick leave, were known about and lobbied about by John and David beforehand, yet had remained in the final wording of the Act. (That century-old hole remains in government statutory sick pay provision today, although trade union lobbying over the years means most employers cover it with their own sick pay provision.)

The final impact of the Act would only be known once the effect could be seen on the ground, in terms of whether it achieved its aim in reducing the number of working-age people claiming Poor Law relief.

Other issues, for example difficulties in administration, would only become clear once the administration of the Act started. John was the first to spot one of the key issues facing the Oddfellows and other friendly societies operating in more than one country across England, Wales and Scotland, known as the 'border difficulty'. The new Act assumed that a person working at a location in, say, Wales, would belong to a friendly society lodge in Wales. While this was often the case, there were many people who moved back and forth across the borders. In border counties like Montgomeryshire, one week a farm labourer might be needed by a farmer in Wales; the next week, they might go to help out a farm down the road which happened to be in England. On the road from Montgomery to the neighbouring town of Bishop's Castle, people would cross the border three times in the space of a few miles.

Having a friendly society account was a bit like having a bank account – you needed to keep paying into the same account in order to build up the benefits you were entitled to. You couldn't just start opening new accounts at random at different branches. So, letting people crossing the border keep their existing friendly society membership was essential.

John first raised the border difficulty at the Oddfellows' national conference in 1912. At the same conference the year before, John had proposed a delegation of Oddfellows going to see the chancellor of the exchequer, Lloyd George, about the administration of the National Insurance Act, yet in the end it could not be arranged due to civil servants' availability. This year, John was determined that a group should go and present their grievances directly to the minister. This was agreed by the conference and John was appointed as part of the deputation from the Oddfellows nationally to meet the chancellor to discuss the border difficulty.

Lloyd George had been the chancellor in Asquith's liberal government since 1908. The reason John kept suggesting going to see him about the Act became clear. This is the most senior position a Welsh person had ever reached in government, and there was a way in through the local MP, David Davies, who was now good friends with Lloyd George. Lloyd George was already a great supporter of the Welsh national TB service initiated by David and John. Therefore he would likely give them a fair hearing.

The deputation to the chancellor of the exchequer took place on 29 July 1912. In the end it was Lloyd George's senior staff who met them, rather than Lloyd George himself. John led the representations, explaining the issues in detail to Lister Stead, permanent secretary to the Treasury – the highest of the chancellor's civil servants.[5]

The chancellor didn't immediately agree to resolve the issue. John kept lobbying at all levels, from the Oddfellows' grassroots members to MPs. In September, John spoke at the National Conference of Friendly Societies for the first time, where all friendly societies met together annually. John raised the issue of the border difficulty and received a lot of support from other delegates at the conference at Newcastle upon Tyne. John's speech was reported in the *Nottingham Evening Post* with the headline 'That Insurance Act! – Friendly Society Complaints':

> Bro. Tomley said the effect of that regulation was the disintegration of every society which had members in each of the four countries. It was only right to say that this clause was introduced into the Bill by an amendment moved by the Chancellor of the Exchequer and carried without debate under the closure, and among 470 amendments passed on one memorable evening in the House of Commons. The effect of this provision would be to make the administration of sickness akin to the red tape work of the Poor Law...[6]

John continued correspondence with the Insurance Commissioners after the visit to the chancellor of the exchequer's office. Eventually his campaigning on the border difficulty was successful: by December 1912, action was being taken in Parliament. An amending Act was promised that would resolve the issue. Everyone breathed a sigh of relief. John's campaign had finally succeeded.[7]

When the amending Act appeared, however, it was not what John and his colleagues had hoped for. While one issue was resolved, another was put in its place. The Welsh Insurance Commissioners were worried about their jobs. If most of the friendly societies were UK wide, they would not have headquarters in Wales, and then the commissioners would have nothing to do. They would be out of a job. So the Welsh Insurance Commissioners decided to change the wording of the amendment, to state that people in Wales would have to join a friendly society with headquarters in Wales. This meant that the Oddfellows and other UK-wide organisations would have to be broken up into separate countries.

John pointed out to everyone the big issue here. While this sounded great from a nationalist point of view, and he himself was a Welsh nationalist, there were times when nationalism was not the best approach. In Wales, a poor country with high unemployment, many young Welsh people were forced to move to England to find work. They would be paying their National Insurance contributions in England, so Wales was short of contributions. This meant the amount of money coming in for National Insurance in Wales was lower than the amount of money going out. The Oddfellows had been operating like this for decades, subsidising the Welsh lodges. If Wales was split out, the Welsh part would go bust and everyone would lose their health insurance benefits they had paid in for.

The Welsh Commissioners did not take this lying down. They fought tooth and nail to discredit John for speaking out, changing their rules so that John was no longer allowed to be employed by both a friendly society and in his role as a local health commissioner, at the National Health Committee at Montgomeryshire County Council. There was an outcry by the Oddfellows as the whole point was that John was a boundary spanner – he knew how both local government and friendly societies work, and the two groups would otherwise be siloed. John was forced to give up his Oddfellows paid role as lodge secretary and local friendly society auditor, although he could continue to volunteer as a member of the Oddfellows' national Investigation Committee.

The political games played by the Welsh Insurance Commissioners continued apace. The Oddfellows' national conference in Aberystwyth in May 1914 heard that they had introduced a new rule for Wales which the Oddfellows' members disagreed with, preventing meeting in pubs. While the Oddfellows preferred other meeting places if possible, in some villages there wasn't anywhere suitable, so it meant the village could no longer have its own branch. In the days before cars, this prevented people claiming their sickness benefits as they could not travel, especially when sick.

To fight against this rule, the Oddfellows' director A.H. Warren went to see Charles Masterman, the minister responsible, 'in his room at the House of Commons, and entered a strong protest on behalf of the Unity at the action of the Commissioners. Mr. Masterman promised that the most careful inquiry should be made into the whole matter.'

The Oddfellows board then arranged a follow-up meeting with the Welsh Insurance Commissioners. During the meeting, the Commissioners gave the Oddfellows board members what were supposedly letters that local Oddfellows branch leaders in Wales had written to the South Wales papers, in support of the new rule, behind the backs of the

Oddfellows board. The *Oddfellows Magazine* reported: 'At the moment the deputation was nonplussed. Several of the Commissioners regarded those communications with great hilarity and laughed at the deputation's confusion.' It then turned out that the local branch leaders had been visited by a member of the Welsh Insurance Commissioners' staff pretending to be a newspaper reporter, who had hoodwinked them into it. In the next article, John got his photo in the magazine again, speaking against the break-up attempt.[8]

Local health commissioners unite

John had realized that to overcome the issues being caused by the National Health Insurance legislation and the Welsh Insurance Commissioners, it was important for all the local health commissioners to band together and have a united approach. To do this, John helped set up the Association of Welsh Insurance Committees. The first meeting was in February 1914, with John on its executive committee. John suggested to add to the aims of the committee 'to secure efficiency and the standardisation of methods and form', and this was included.

Although John may have been forced by the Welsh Insurance Commissioners to give up his paid Oddfellows role as lodge secretary, he had soon picked up two new roles. He had become a member of the National Health Insurance Advisory Committee for Wales, a UK government-level committee, managed by the chancellor of the exchequer's office. This was a precursor to his later work on similar Ministry of Health committees – at the time, the Ministry of Health had not yet been set up (this would happen in 1919). It is likely that John had been appointed by Lloyd George after leading the Oddfellows delegation, perhaps after a suggestion by David Davies to his friend the Welsh Wizard.[9] John was on this committee as a friendly society representative for the Oddfellows. Another member of the committee who had been appointed at the same time was Samuel Filer from Tredegar, representing the Medical Aid societies, the local friendly societies in South Wales and Monmouthshire. It is likely that Samuel came from the Tredegar Medical Aid Society, where Nye Bevan would later join the board.

The other new role was John's first international one. The Association of Welsh Insurance Committees appointed John as one of the five representatives of Wales on the International Federation of Insurance Committees. Now John would be able to learn more about the new state health and unemployment insurance systems in other countries such as Germany and France.[10]

On the facing page of the *Oddfellows Magazine* article mentioning John's two new roles, there was a request for information about industrial life assurance to the Oddfellows members from Sidney Webb from the Fabian Society's Fabian Research Department – the Fabian Society was a radical socialist group connected to the founding of the Labour Party, and Webb had been co-founder of the London School of Economics back in 1895. Sidney Webb asked the same question the Oddfellows were asking about private versus state and mutual society provision: 'We want to know why millions of poor people prefer the expensive policies of the companies to the cheaper policies of the Post Office.'[11]

The Oddfellows worked closely with the Fabians for many years. Beatrice Webb and her husband Sidney were instrumental in introducing William Beveridge to social policy research work in the East End of London. William Beveridge ended up staying with the Liberal Party, while the Webbs went on to help found the Labour Party.

John continued to campaign against the new amended legislation, writing to the papers and making speeches decrying the breaking-up attempt by the government. Eventually John was successful and there was another new amendment agreed to the Act to sort it out.

Over the next decade, John continued his lobbying. As well as the issues mentioned above, there were numerous other holes in the Act. It did not cover death benefit, so widows and orphans did not receive anything if their breadwinner died, and family members struggled to pay for funerals. John pointed out that the new equivalent scheme in Germany included both death and accident benefits.

In September 1913, John spoke at the National Conference of Friendly Societies at the Hearts of Oak offices in London, on the subject of the border difficulty. The conference at that time represented just over four million adult members in the UK. At a later session in the conference, the president that year, A.H. Warren, said 'they did not desire that national insurance should turn us into a nation of men and women who were grandmothered into the world, and grandmothered through the world, and grandmothered out of the world. That was to say, they did not want the rising generation to take national insurance as the standard of all that was required from them.'[12]

Around the same time, John attended an Oddfellows meeting at Abergavenny where the meeting opposed a state medical service. Fortunately for us, the rising generation like John had different views.

They wanted everyone to have the security of a national health service and universal welfare, from the cradle to the grave.

Photo opportunities

In May 1912, John had been at the Oddfellows' Annual Moveable Conference in Nottingham. After standing for a place for several years running, for the first time John finally won enough votes to become one of the ten Oddfellows representatives to the National Conference of Friendly Societies. He also became captain of the Cosmopolitan Party, one of the Oddfellows' social groups, replacing the former captain who had just been elected as deputy grand master of the Oddfellows. John was now rubbing shoulders with the people at the top of the friendly society. He got his photo in the magazine again too – as one of the younger men, this was probably the Edwardian friendly society equivalent of being a magazine pin-up.[13]

The same magazine also reported that John's Montgomery district of Oddfellows had appointed a ladies' committee to draft rules for the new female lodges being set up, so that more women could become members. Sidney Pryce's wife Mary was one of the committee members, implying that she was particularly keen on equal rights for women.

In January 1913, the *Oddfellows Magazine* reported that John had been nominated by Montgomeryshire District to stand for the directorate as well as his existing Investigation Committee role. Clearly he had impressed enough people with his successful lobbying for the change in legislation on the border difficulty.[14]

In March, John's father Robert died. He had just lived long enough to see John lecturing on the new National Health Insurance, managing to get legislation changed and standing for the Oddfellows directorate – all his dreams for what his son might achieve had been fulfilled.[15]

By 1913, John and his wife Edith had moved house to Plas Du on Old Gaol Road in Montgomery, a larger house to accommodate their growing family now they had three children.[16] Their first home at 3 Alexandria Terrace on Chirbury Road had looked very attractive, yet from the council meeting minutes it turned out it was actually built on the old town cess pool – basically a big open sewer – so it may not have been the most sanitary place to live. This may be why they had moved to Plas Du. They must have moved to The Hollies quite soon after, buying it from the Farmer sisters, the suffragettes.

In May 1913, John spoke several times at the Oddfellows' Annual Moveable Conference in Scarborough, reported again in the *Oddfellows Magazine*, including on the questions of women members, valuations for National Insurance members, and pressing for copies of the Oddfellows' general rules in Welsh so that members could properly understand them.

In the first article, John got his photo printed yet again. The Oddfellows now had a lot more female members thanks to John's efforts, so I hope his fans appreciated the photo of the handsome young man who was publicly saying he believed in votes for women, at a time when this was highly controversial. Had he been inspired by a recent chat with the Farmer sisters perhaps?

John said that

> if they admitted a female as a member to a lodge, they must admit that female member to the meeting of the lodge. It seemed to him, if a female could attend any meeting for the payment of her contributions to the lodge, she could attend every meeting for the good of her lodge. They did not believe in taxation without representation. They believed, so far as Oddfellows were concerned, in votes for women.

His proposal was successfully carried.[17]

The following year, in May 1914, the annual conference was in the Pier Pavilion at Aberystwyth, in mid Wales. Unlike the more staid civil servants and government committees, the friendly societies were working men's movements and there was more banter. John had to move seamlessly between these different worlds and try to persuade everyone to work together, while upholding his own professional standards as a member of the legal profession.

The time came for the conference delegates to vote for the design for the almanack, an annual book sent to Oddfellows members. Three designs were presented, titled 'Friendship', 'Love', and 'Truth', with symbols of England, Scotland and Ireland. John spoke up, objecting to the designs as they did not contain any symbols of Wales, such as leeks. 'Were they... going to adopt a design that did not contain symbolic representation of the Principality? (Applause.)' The Grand Master didn't miss a beat. He asked the person presenting the designs, 'Bro. Appleyard, what are you going to do with the leek?' Much laughter ensued and John got his wish.[18]

The real reason for the CBE

In July 1914, the First World War started and most normal business was put on hold to assist with the war effort. John worked hard during the First World War, yet there are no records of his contribution in the newspapers as it was confidential war work. During my recent discoveries about John Tomley's contribution in life, I was surprised when my uncle told me that, contrary to my granny's claim, 'he didn't get a CBE for setting up the NHS in 1948, that was earlier'. What? So he did something else that was worth a CBE too? What was that?

The only mention in the newspapers is eight years later, in 1922, when he received a CBE for this and other work he had done before the war and is mentioned in a series on 'Prominent Men in Mid-Wales: 'When, during the war, the heaviness of casualties called for joint hospital arrangements to be made in North Wales, Mr Tomley was at once chosen as Chairman of the Joint Hospital Committee.'[19]

John had been tasked with running all hospital services for the whole of the North Wales region, when they needed to work together to cope with the casualties coming in from the battlefields like the Somme in France. This region probably meant the top half of Wales, from Montgomeryshire to Deeside. Hospitals at this time were independent and did not usually work with each other, yet the emergency war situation meant they were forced to temporarily. John would have been a natural choice for this role as he already had experience of running the WNMA's national TB service for Wales, as well as county health services as a local health commissioner. The First World War would prove crucial in proving that hospitals could work together on a national basis – again something prefiguring the NHS.

After the WNMA had been created as the first ever national health service, the hospitals John led in the First World War were effectively the second version of a national health service. Yet this learning would be ignored immediately after the war because of the country's overstretched finances. It would take both the Welsh TB Inquiry report in 1939, followed by the same system being set up again for the Second World War – the third national health service – to remind everyone that it had worked well. Then today's NHS would finally be set up in 1948. So our NHS was not the first national health service as we often think today, but in fact the fourth version of a national health service.

In 1914 when war broke out, within weeks casualties were flooding back to the UK from France. North Wales was a good place for military casualties as it was close to the port of Liverpool, so people could be transported there by boat. There was also plenty of space there. There were far too many patients for the existing military hospitals. The government had to organise for patients to be cared for in workhouses and voluntary hospitals. The hospital services at the time were 'uncoordinated and haphazard' so it was a major task to bring them together. The hospitals agreed to do this. Yet it soon proved to be a heavy burden, both in terms of staff time and effort and shortfalls in the War Office grants, which did not cover the full costs of care, causing many hospitals to end the war in deficit.[20] John had to work hard to bring everyone together in North Wales to overcome these issues and provide the best possible care.

After people injured in the war had recovered in hospital, there were two options. People who were fully fit and could work and fight again would be sent home for a rest before potentially being sent back out to the battlefields. Yet many people did not fully recover. Many people had permanent physical injuries, such as losing a limb, or pain from embedded shrapnel. The next logical stage for this was obvious, that people with disabilities needed to be supported to be rehabilitated so that they could return home and make a living for themselves where possible. Many people in this situation could no longer do their old job due to their disability, so they needed to be retrained and find new employment. People also needed war pensions to support them and their families for the rest of their lives if they were no longer able to earn a full wage.

John therefore took on a second role too, as chairman of the North Wales Joint Disablements Committee, leading on rehabilitation and pensions for the region.[21]

As John explained in speeches:

> He hoped they would take every possible interest in these disabled men as they returned, as strong and active committees existed to provide for the treatment, training, and employment of disabled men. No one wished to see these brave fellows who had given their best for their country to be penalised in any way by their service in the King's uniform.[22]

And he upheld that the government should

> provide training for men disabled from following their previous employment. It is undesirable for such men to get into 'blind-alley' occupations which they may lose after the war. Men being trained will have travelling expenses paid, be

> boarded or billeted at the expense of the State, wives and families continue to receive their allowances, and men be granted a bonus of 5s. per week at the conclusion of training. Whatever a man may be able to earn as a result of training, his pension will not be affected. [23]

As a result of these roles John had 'a position of honourable distinction in the working of two important Acts of Parliament... The initial shaping of the administration of the War Pensions Acts and orders not only in Montgomeryshire but also – in certain branches of work – in the six counties of North Wales, was in a large measure, Mr Tomley's work.'[24] This refers to the War Pensions Acts 1915–1921, a series of Acts of Parliament introducing state war pensions for First World War casualties and their dependants. John ensured that pensions were generous, and all the needs of disabled soldiers were dealt with by one government department, the Ministry of Pensions, rather than several, making it much fairer and more efficient. It was not necessary for a soldier to have seen active service – for example many people had contracted diseases like TB during their military training and would still be eligible for pensions.

In November 1916, John was also elected President of the Association of Welsh Insurance Committees, which he had helped set up following the issues with the National Insurance Act legislation and the Welsh Insurance Commissioners. This was his first national leadership role.

The Oddfellows in wartime

John continued to attend the Oddfellows conferences and the National Conference of Friendly Societies during the First World War.

In May 1915, the Annual Moveable Conference was held in the Manchester Free Trade Hall. John was appointed vice-chair of the Oddfellows' Investigation Committee, and was involved in discussions on a doctor preparing a medical handbook for local officers of the society and the doctor's recommendation to use the name of the disease rather than symptoms on medical certificates.

By the time war conscription started in January 1916, John was 42, just over the limit. He must have felt frustrated to see his army reserve colleagues leaving without him. David Davies, a few years younger than John, stayed in his MP role but saw action in France as commander of the

14th Royal Welch Fusiliers, being made a major. In July 1916 he returned to serve as Lloyd George's parliamentary secretary, the latter becoming prime minister that December. However, they were soon to fall out. Lloyd George sacked David in June 1917, and thereafter David became an outspoken critic of his former friend.

In October 1916, John represented the Oddfellows at the National Conference of Friendly Societies. After being ruled 'out of order' when he spoke about TB the previous year, this time he managed to get a resolution for friendly societies to put pressure on local authorities to reduce TB by removing 'the insanitary conditions with which so many sufferers from tuberculosis are surrounded'. The resolution was carried.[25]

A year later, John attended a special National Conference of Friendly Societies, which was held to discuss the government's proposal to create a minister of health for the first time. Despite some misgivings that the government was trying to take over the friendly societies' work, it was decided by the conference to support the government's proposal. This is when the post which would later be held by Nye Bevan was first created.

To ensure the government could afford the war pensions and the new Ministry of Health, John urged the friendly societies at the conference to avoid making any further claims on government funding for death liabilities from war. The cost of a lifetime pension for a disabled soldier, which John was probably involved in negotiating and the government had now agreed to pay, was much more than the funeral cost for a soldier who had died, which the friendly society had to pay. For every soldier who died, many more were disabled. So the largest cost for the friendly societies had been funded.

Chair of the Oddfellows Investigation Committee

After the war, in May 1919 John was at the Oddfellows' Annual Moveable Conference in Douglas. He had now been promoted to chair of the Investigation Committee. He reported a higher number than usual of cases of hardship that had not been relieved by grants from local lodges, due to the effects of the war. John asked the wider question of whether old-age pensions were adequate, highlighted by the large number of grant applications. State pension rates had only increased from 5s. to 7s. 6d. per week over the decade since they had been introduced, and were now well behind inflation so many pensioners were unable to cover their essential living costs. In many cases they could not award hardship grants under a certain amount, because whatever the Oddfellows gave would be clawed back from people's state pensions.

Sir Alfred Warren MP enthusiastically supported John's proposal for the Manchester Unity board of directors 'to make urgent and immediate representation to the Government to increase the present maximum old-age pension to at least 10s. per week'. John had probably lined up Warren to support this in advance. John explained:

> The whole question of the amount of old-age pensions was being considered by a special Government Department, and it was incumbent upon the Unity to make representations as to the desirability of increasing the grant, in view of the circumstances of the present day. They did not consider that they were asking for any charity dole; they were acting as the mouthpiece of these old-age pensioners who had no organization of their own. There must be thousands of brethren in the Unity whose circumstances were only slightly better than those to whom grants had been made.

In July, John himself was one of the experts invited to give evidence to the government Select Committee looking at old-age pensions, chaired by Sir Ryland Adkins, a Liberal MP for Lancashire. Arnold Rowntree MP, nephew of chocolate manufacturer and philanthropist Joseph Rowntree, was also on the panel.

John pushed for a rate of 15s. per week. He explained that two-thirds of the people over 70 in Montgomeryshire met the means test to be eligible for an old-age pension, and of those, around a third of people had no other means of support. Therefore, the pension rate needed to be set high enough to buy essentials, and essentials had increased in price due to the war. 'Just think of what food alone will cost, apart from what coal will cost the poor people this winter.' People who had kept pigs and poultry at home before the war, which had helped them be more self-sufficient, could no longer afford the animal food.

The Oddfellows nationally had supported the increase to at least 10s. at their recent annual conference. After the Old-Age Pensions Act had originally been passed, the Oddfellows had no cases of people with an old-age pension who needed extra financial support. Now, around a quarter of hardship grant claims were from people who already received an old-age pension.

People were unwilling to claim Poor Law relief to supplement their pensions. John explained to the committee:

> We come from the Lloyd George country and the pension is spoken of as the Lloyd George money. It is the Lloyd George 5s. to these people. I do not know whether you are acquainted with Wales. It means a good deal to them. If you called it anything else, say poor-rate money, it would not have the same halo round it as at present... If it comes under the Poor Law you cannot diminish the taint that is associated with the Poor Law.

Arnold Rowntree asked, 'You want the pension which is given to the poorest type of person to be sufficient to keep that person?' John replied 'Yes', having also made the point 'There ought to be enough to keep body and soul alive.'

John also pushed for old-age pensions to start at 65 instead of 70, as many people aged 65 to 70 were unable to work due to ill health yet were too young to claim a pension, so were forced to rely on Poor Law relief and the workhouses.[26]

By the following year, there had been two very welcome breakthroughs thanks to the work of John and others. Pensions had been increased from 7s. 6d. to 10s. per week, and pensioners would no longer be disqualified for receiving Poor Law relief. This meant the very poorest people would now have the benefit of a pension.[27]

John had continued to attend the National Conference of Friendly Societies each year. In September 1919, John was speaking at the conference in Cardiff, calling for an inquiry into industrial insurance – the same issue Sidney Webb of the Fabians was working on.[28] There was also a possible new appointment for John discussed. He was nominated to the new Ministry of Health's Advisory Consultative Councils.[29]

Later, after the conference, there is a report of who had ended up on the Ministry of Health committee. John's name, despite being submitted, was left off – a 'regrettable omission' of someone 'who has done much valuable work in connection with the administration of National Insurance in Wales'. John was already unpopular with the Welsh commissioners for his work on the border difficulty which could have put them out of a job, and now had refused to accept amalgamation of the rural branches. The commissioners had clearly chosen people who would be less likely to fight them.[30]

In October 1919, the discussion about TB continued at the Association of Welsh Insurance Committees' annual conference at Swansea. The president, Mr J.W. Jones, praised the work of the Welsh National Memorial Association. During the war, the WNMA's work had more than quadrupled, from running 235 hospital and sanatoria beds in July 1914, to running 1,067 beds in July 1919. Over 12,000 patients per year were now being seen.[31] The Ministry of Health's powers were being increased, which meant that they might be able to get rid of the slums which were making TB efforts ineffective.

John submitted the annual report, which explained that there was a lack of training, meaning special exercise to get rid of TB for consumptive soldiers. *The Western Mail* reported:

> Although the subject had been brought up two years ago, the situation was still terrible. Those who had contracted the disease in the Army and Navy had not been provided with the training for which they had been pleading; men who had thrown up occupations to fight for their country were left without provision for this concurrent treatment. He condemned this as a positive scandal.[32]

By the time of the same conference the following year (October 1920) there had been no further movement on the issue. The Oddfellows, too, had been rebuffed when they tried to meet with the government to ask for help with the costs of supporting members who had been in the war. David Davies' pre-war cosy relationship with Lloyd George was no more. John could therefore do very little of political influence through working with David at this time. Fortunately, John now had his own political contacts.

In September 1921, more doom and gloom filled the national press, yet there could still be lighter moments. The *Daily News* of 28 September carried a range of headlines on its front page: 'Unemployment an appalling problem', 'Europe's peril'… But there was also a 'Strange story about a Welsh grave'. Exactly a century before, a highwayman called John Newton Davies was hanged in Montgomery and on the scaffold declared he was innocent, and no grass would grow on his grave for a century, a prophecy which apparently had held true. The story reached the papers thanks to one John Tomley, who as a council employee was responsible for promoting the area and had been writing tourism articles in the newspaper for many years. Thereafter the site received many visitors and despite the economic downturn, this meant local businesses in Montgomery were doing well out of them. John himself took a party of historians around the Robber's Grave and Montgomery Castle, where he gave them a talk on the castle's history, which became a booklet, 'The Castle of Montgomery', sold locally by the *Montgomery Express* for only sixpence and advertised as 'a valuable brochure'.

In the meantime, in August 1921, John's 16-year-old daughter Doris had a lucky escape at Lymore Hall, neglected for years by the Earl of Powis, after the floor collapsed. The *Montgomeryshire Express* reported:

> A most untoward accident, fortunately unattended by fatal consequences, occurred at the bazaar and fete held at Lymore Hall, Montgomery, on Thursday last... The business of the bazaar was in full swing... a laughing, gaily chatting throng. Suddenly, without any audible premonitary symptoms, a knot of guests was observed to disappear outright.
>
> The polished oak floor on which they were seen to stand had disappeared over a space of about twelve feet by six feet. It had all happened almost noiselessly, and those standing in the immediate neighbourhood were for the moment petrified... With the people who fell into the vault was the fancy stall over which Miss Doris Tomley presided. The young lady, fortunately, did not accompany her stand in its downward track, but was left standing on the edge of the chasm. The Earl of Powis was at the time talking to the Rector of Montgomery. Lord Powis disappeared, but the Rector was left on the solid floor. The Earl escaped with very slight injuries, as also did his agent, Mr J. Edmonds, who when in the depths found himself almost inextricably mixed with the fancy goods of Miss Tomley's stall.[33]

The 17 people who fell 12 feet through the floor with the Earl of Powis also included J. D. K. Lloyd's parents, and a female journalist from the *County Times*. Fortunately, there were no serious injuries. John's friend Robert Bunner, who supplied the local building trade, was particularly vocal on the subject of the Earl of Powis's lack of maintenance skills. Lymore Hall was demolished soon afterwards. The floor collapse incident went down in folk memory in Montgomery. My dad and his brothers (who were born in Montgomery two decades later) often used Lymore as an example to warn us about the importance of home maintenance.

David Davies, meanwhile, was now focusing on his role as owner of Ocean Coal Company, installing the first pithead baths in South Wales mines and the second to be installed in Britain, as well as rolling out social housing, old age pensions and recreational associations for his own mine and railway workers. Soon his railways would be amalgamated with Great Western Railways and David would become a director of GWR.[34]

Friendly societies propose a national health service

In September 1921, John attended the National Conference of Friendly Societies in Bournemouth, where the president, Bro. T. Lewis, Hearts of Oak, suggested a national health service should be set up. The friendly societies

> ought to concentrate their attention upon securing a thorough, all-embracing public health service under the Ministry of Health. This, of course, would include the public medical service, which they had demanded on many occasions.
>
> It is patent, I think, that we are not getting the value for the enormous sum paid to the medical profession – a total nearly as great as the amount spent on sickness, disablement and maternity benefits. The economists in the House of Commons, when discussing the administration of health insurance, should bear this point in mind...
>
> A proper medical service must be co-ordinated with hospitals, nursing and other services. A fine nucleus already exists in the present public health services, and it is in the extension of these that we must look for the solution of the preventative side of our work.

Lewis affirmed the importance of prevention being better than cure for illnesses such as TB, and the role of housing and pensions in that. He called for a 'really efficient medical service' and there was criticism from his fellows that doctors had prospered while also moving away to be 'miles from their clients': 'If anybody had done well out of the Insurance Act it was the doctors'. A Mr G. Belsten, also from Hearts of Oak, observed:

> In 1915, the medical men in this country had taken within a few hundred pounds as much as the people who had received

69

benefit under the Insurance Act. The doctors had nearly £5,000,000, and the benefit in the ordinary way ran to a little over £5,000,000.

The Rev. F. Ranking, National Catholic Benefit Society, pointed out that the difficulty was the patients, unfortunately, were not willing to complain, because they were afraid of what the doctors might do afterwards.[35]

Later in the conference, Sir Alfred Warren, the parliamentary agent, warned the conference about the forthcoming economy drive, met with suspicion by the Oddfellows attending. 'They were aware of the wave of economy. It was called the economy stunt, and they knew how it was being engineered.'[36]

This is the exact issue that the NHS and welfare state faces today. Whenever calls are made for proper funding to fill the holes in services that have opened up due to budget cuts since the 1970s, just as things start to gain momentum, resistance is organized. Certain politicians tell us that the NHS is very inefficient and if it was just run more efficiently, there would be no need for any more money, so it is not worth giving extra funding. In fact, the NHS should be able to make do with less. This confuses the public, and so we stop asking.

Soon after the Bournemouth conference in 1921, it was reported that the doctors had been challenged on their high fees. The panel doctors' conference agreed with Sir Alfred Mond, minister of health, to accept a reduction in their fees from 11s. to 9s. per patient, on patriotic grounds and grounds of public economy.

The same year, John was at a special meeting of the National Conference of Friendly Societies where there was a threat to John's work with David at the WNMA. A government efficiency drive meant that TB sanatorium benefit had been deleted from the Amended National Health Insurance Bill. John organized action against this proposal by all the insurance committees in Wales.[37] His campaign was successful and the sanatorium benefit was kept.

In May 1922, John attended the Oddfellows' annual conference at Guernsey, again chairing the Investigation Committee. He launched the Orphan Gift Fund, a hardship grant fund for children orphaned in the war or for other reasons, which still exists today – I'm a member of the Oddfellows myself so it is available to my daughter. John had two photos this time, one by himself as usual (pre-war) and one with the rest of the Investigation Committee (post war, with markedly less hair – his pin-up days were now behind him, as comes to us all).[38]

Role under threat

After his sterling war service and CBE, what thanks did John get? By February 1922, his role on the Welsh War Pensions Committee was under threat and might be taken over by a civil servant parachuted in from London. A newspaper report headed 'Welsh pensions positions: jobs for civil servants from London?' reported:

> It was stated at the meeting of the Montgomeryshire War Pensions Committee, at Newtown, on Wednesday, that it was quite possible the Ministry were contemplating the placing of Civil servants from London in the secretarial positions in Wales under the new Pensions Act of 1921.
> Mr J. Griffiths, the committee's representative on the Welsh Regional Council, said that these men would be most probably inefficient compared with those who had done the work up to the present, and would lack local ... The result would be that the ex-service men would be placed under the power of men with no intimate knowledge of their cases.
> A strong resolution was passed urging the Ministry to retain the services of Mr J. E. Tomley, the secretary of the Montgomeryshire committee.[39]

August 1922 brought some much-needed lighter relief for John, as he was appointed vice-president of the newly established Central Wales National Football League, with David Davies as president. After playing football himself and captaining the local team at Montgomery, John had continued as a referee and then became chairman of Division III of the Central Wales section of the Welsh League.[40]

The Geddes Axe

In September 1922, John attended the next National Conference of Friendly Societies, in Cheltenham. A new threat was on the horizon for health, National Insurance and pensions: the Geddes Axe. The cost-saving drive mentioned the year before had begun, with recommendations made by a Committee on National Expenditure chaired by Sir Eric Geddes, who had been director-general of munitions and railways in the First World War.

The *Oddfellows Magazine* reported:

> The President [Councillor G.F. Kelly, Leeds, Ancient Order of Foresters] said he felt they were passing through a perilous period... The Geddes Axe, being a popular weapon, all sorts and conditions of men had come under its powerful blows. The suggested increase of National Insurance contributions was soon dropped, but [others were] not so easily given up...
>
> With regard to tuberculosis, there had been great promises but very few of these had been fulfilled. This disease was largely due to ignorance and poverty. When they urged upon the Ministry of Health the necessity that adequate provision should be made for the dependants of afflicted persons they were at once referred to the Poor Law, as there were no hopes of any assistance from the Treasury. Personally, he was of opinion this dreadful scourge should be attacked at its source. In his judgement the housing of the people was where the remedy should be sought...
>
> On the question of old age pensions they had been passing pious resolutions for years, and it was time they entered with greater force into the political arena...
>
> The question of medical benefit from the inception of the Insurance Act had been a troublesome one to all concerned. Doctors and approved societies were not yet satisfied with the service... The medical profession was making rash statements and giving out wholesale threats. He ventured to suggest to the Minister of Health that he would be well advised to hand over to the approved societies the medical benefits as a whole. He was fully persuaded this could be done and the insured person better served. By such a process the insurance committees could be scrapped and a huge sum of money saved to the country.[41]

In the end the £87 million of economies proposed by Geddes were reduced to £52 million, but nonetheless spending on social issues such as education, health, housing, pensions and unemployment fell by almost 12 per cent between 1920–1 and 1922–3, and a further 4 per cent the year after. For John and his fellow reformers, there would clearly be plenty of challenges ahead.

Chapter 4

'The Busy Man'
1923–1930

The Welsh National Memorial Association opened its first children's hospital for TB, St Bride's Hospital in Pembrokeshire, in June 1923. The building, St Bride's Castle, was previously known as the Kensington Hospital and had been purchased from Lord Kensington by the WNMA. The hospital would now be used as a home for children with surgical tuberculosis.

Many people attended the opening, including John Tomley, doctors from all over Wales and England, and John Rowland from the Welsh Board of Health. David Davies was there with his new second wife Henrietta, after his first wife Amy had died in 1918 from a tropical illness she had picked up on their honeymoon in 1910. Henrietta received the key from Mr E.W.G. Richards, the architect, and formally declared the hospital open.

Sir John Lynn-Thomas, a well-known surgeon, said that 'since the foundation of the association, thirteen years ago, 30,000 patients had been treated at the different institutions. They had the finest organisation in the world to combat the disease, and in spite of the war they had made great strides'. Dr Llew Williams, chief medical officer of the Welsh Board of Health, said 'thanks to the munificence of the Llandinam family [Llandinam was David Davies' family home], the memorial to the late King Edward had become a fact; and that day was opened and established for the first time a hospital for the treatment of tubercular children.'[1]

Yet TB was still far from being eradicated. In early 1923, the *Oddfellows Magazine* reported on the latest statistics:

> A MOST disquieting statement as to the greater prevalence of tuberculosis in rural than in industrial areas was made at the annual meeting of the Montgomery district by Bro. J.E. Tomley... Attention was drawn to the lack of facilities for disinfection, the miserable housing conditions, ignorance of people as to obtaining treatment in early stages of the disease, and laxity in notification to the tuberculosis physician. It was suggested that the local education authority should lay special stress on the teaching of hygiene, and that

the attention of doctors should be drawn to the importance of referring suspicious cases to the tuberculosis physician...

Bro. J.E. Tomley said the incidence of tuberculosis in country districts was about 6 to 4 compared with urban areas... They had a greater proportion of tuberculosis in North Wales than in South Wales, but in the South Wales area there was a greater proportion of fatal cases. The result was that they in North Wales had a larger proportion of continuing cases, consequently remaining longer on the funds, and incidentally tuberculosis cases cost half as much again per member as in South Wales...

Dr. Owen Morris, in the course of his address, said a campaign against tuberculosis would also stamp out many other diseases. The chief thing they should look after was good food and that involved the keeping up of wages...

The best thing they could do was to teach the people preventive measures, and train them to take more heed to doctors' advice. Tuberculosis never ran in families; it probably was in their blankets or in their carpets...[2]

Oddfellows trustee

John continued to chair the Oddfellows' Investigation Committee for many years. He was involved in further political wrangling with the government, of course.

In 1923, he attended the National Conference of Friendly Societies in Aberystwyth. The Geddes Axe had fallen and the government was in no mood for spending. There was little to report: there was nothing much that could be fought for now, in terms of improvements to health and social security. It was reported the hospital accommodation was inadequate with long waiting lists everywhere, and doctors were fighting friendly societies to demand that they had first call on the funds, i.e., that doctor's bills should take precedence over paying amounts to sick members to cover their living costs. There was a suggestion that TB patients in sanatoria should pay a means-tested charge, which John pointed out was unfair when they were not earning. It might also deter people seeking help, and therefore make them more likely to infect other people.[3]

A year later, at the conference in Folkestone, John's committee 'recommended the accepting of the financial liability for the maintenance of 65 orphans, children of deceased members, to 16 years of age, at a cost to the orphan fund of £14,000':

> Mr J.E. Tomley (Montgomery), in moving the adoption of the Committee's recommendation, described it as one of the most magnificent acts in the history of Oddfellowship. These little ones would bless the day on which their parents joined the society.[4]

As well as widowed mothers' pensions, another item discussed at the same meeting was the 'recurring spasm' of panel doctors' fees. The doctors were asking for an increase in their pay which was more than the increase in state funding. The doctors also said they would work for friendly societies but not for the state. This is why the full NHS was not set up until many years later.

The final session of the Oddfellows' annual conference in July 1924 led to a further development in John's career, when he had the chance to stand for election for a trustee role.[5] In the voting, John and Sir Alfred Warren were the only two candidates left in the final round for one seat on the board. John had 256 votes in the previous round, and Warren had 222. Sir Alfred Warren was much older and more experienced than John. He had been an MP and was past grand master of the Unity and president of the National Conference of Friendly Societies. Yet he stood aside for John, who was duly elected as a trustee.[6]

John shared his thoughts for the future at a local Oddfellows meeting:

> Bro. Tomley said they were, no doubt, on the threshold of a new era in the work of the Society. Parliament would consider new arrangements in National Insurance and public assistance generally. The change in old age pensions had abolished assistance from Friendly Societies as a disqualification, and it was evidently in the minds of the statesmen that there should be a contributory scheme of old age pensions, mothers' pensions, and national insurance. He could not see any objection to such a scheme if it was contributory, and this would dispose of any disqualification. The mothers and children of the country had up to the present been neglected in the provisions of the Insurance Acts. The commission which was now sitting to consider possible extensions of those Acts would require evidence

from Friendly Societies, and he was glad to know that active
steps were being taken to supply evidence from Wales.[7]

In September, he attended the National Conference of Friendly Societies in Oxford. Panel doctors remained an issue and the minister of health had therefore set up a Royal Commission to enquire into the working of the National Health Insurance Acts, yet, despite promises, neglected to put anyone 'having a practical knowledge of the administration of the acts' (i.e. friendly society officers) on the committee. The conference committee had complained to the prime minister, the minister of health and the press.

John also explained that the WNMA had been able to keep TB sanatorium treatment free from any means-tested payments for patients, while England was protesting about fees having been forced on them. The WNMA had achieved a huge amount since its creation in 1910. Hospital beds had increased from 23 in 1912 to over 1,000 in 1926.[8]

The same *Oddfellows Magazine* reports that John hosted the grand master at Montgomery for the 93rd anniversary of their lodge in October 1924. John explained that the lodge now had around £10,000 in funds, had been able to afford dental treatment for their members, and they were now living longer too. John's wife, Edith, presented the grand master and his wife with a pair of locally made candlesticks. The grand master congratulated John on the lodge's work and his work, and said Montgomery was one of the brightest spots in the Unity. Music afterwards included 'gramophone selections' by Miss Tomley, one of John's daughters – the newfangled gramophone had found its way to Montgomery.

John also now chaired what had been the Three Counties Conference, which now acknowledged Wales – it had become the Four Counties Conference, for Cheshire, Stafford, Salop [Shropshire] and Montgomery.[9]

In May 1925, John addressed an Oddfellows' conference at Burslem, explaining 'the pension proposals embodied in Mr Winston Churchill's Budget' – another step forward for social security. The year before, John had also written an article explaining the proposals to the public in the *Montgomeryshire Express* newspaper.[10]

Churchill had recently re-joined the Conservative Party after twenty years with the Liberals and had been appointed chancellor of the exchequer. Pensions had been introduced for widows and orphans for the first time. As usual, there were large holes in the provision: the pensions were only for widows only of insured men who had died, and widows only received pensions until the children reached age 14 – the widow then had to find work to support herself. Old-age pensions had now been brought forward to start at age 65 instead of age 70. The basic widow's pension and old-age pension was still 10s. per week – again, it had not increased in line with inflation for the past few years. John also contributed to discussions on this at the Oddfellows' conference in Bournemouth in May 1925, and wrote an article about it in the same magazine with explanatory notes and examples to help the local branches who needed to make sense of the provisions.[11]

At the same conference, John made sure the Orphan Gift Fund continued to age 16, not just age 14 when state support stopped (which prevented orphans continuing their education as they were forced to go to work). The Investigation Committee also had another photo, this time in a slightly less formal pose and looking somewhat like *Reservoir Dogs*...

John spoke at the Oddfellows' Montgomery District annual meeting at the Free Library, Newtown in January 1926 and discussed dental treatment and holes remaining in social security provision for widows again. A colleague reported that David Davies had been lobbying the minister of health about 'the position of persons not insured with incomes comparable with those of people coming under the Act, and stating that they had been left out'. The minister 'apparently recognized the injustice, and from the views expressed they might expect further legislation on the subject'. As ever, Brother Tomley said:

> There was every reason for persisting on behalf of the widows and orphans who were shut out, and it was their duty to their dead brothers and their widows and orphans to insist that the Government should make the same provision for one class as they did for another.[12]

Around this time, everyone in the country was becoming more and more frustrated at the lack of protection for workers suffering after the First World War and now affected by government cuts, resulting in the General Strike of 1.7 million workers, particularly transport and heavy industry, from 4 to 12 May 1926. The purpose of the strike was to support coal miners who were being asked to work longer hours for less pay. The miners' slogan was 'Not a penny off the pay, not a minute on the day'. David Davies supported the miners' call for a 7-hour working day, despite being one of the largest mine owners himself, campaigning against the 'evil spirit which appears to befog every utterance of the coal owners'.[13]

Despite being a huge strike, the General Strike was ultimately unsuccessful, and austerity measures were introduced, threatening the health and social security provision which had been so hard won over the past two decades. John spoke against austerity at an Oddfellows meeting:

> Bro. J. E. Tomley... spoke on the Economy Act... Their Board of Directors were strenuously opposing the measure which would take 2¾ million yearly from the Government contribution to the benefits of the insured population...
> Sir Alfred Warren said the Economy Bill would mean that that which they were hoping to do in getting additional benefits to insured persons would be put back for an indefinite period.[14]

The National Conference of Friendly Societies at Bath in September was dominated by resolutions of protest against the Economy Act with its reduction of the state contribution for National Insurance members from two-ninths to one-seventh. John joined in, speaking against the Economy Act again. As the conference president put it:

> Recent legislation had shown the fallacy of relying upon Government-controlled schemes which could be changed and varied to meet the wishes of a political party when the Government of its choice was in power. The passing of the so-called Economy Act had created a feeling of insecurity and instability in regard to State insurance.[15]

At the Oddfellows' national conference at Great Yarmouth in June 1927, there was some good news – the Investigation Committee reported 'evidence of greater liberality on the part of Poor Law guardians. Frequently they had had to deplore the lack of sympathy shown by those bodies, and they were glad to see the change of feeling.' Yet the issues with many professions and their families being left out of health and social security continued. For the additional benefits the Oddfellows tried to distribute when there was a surplus on the National Insurance scheme, such as dental treatment, the ministry officials had stopped many applications and now said the maximum extra that could be given was 1s., regardless of people's actual needs or circumstances.[16]

In April 1928, John hosted the grand master that year, Bro. Herbert White, and his wife for a holiday in Wales for a few days. John's son Edward, now aged 18, my grandfather, was initiated into the Oddfellows. John must have recently got a car and Edward had now learned to drive. 'Bro. Edward Tomley and Miss Doris Tomley conducted the Grand Master through the regions of mountain, vale and river which characterise one of the most beautiful regions in Great Britain.'[17] This sounds like John let Edward drive the grand master about, perhaps a rather risky decision given Edward's passion for driving fast. Perhaps older sister Doris was keeping an eye on him.

This reminds me of something my granny said to me when I was learning to drive. Like her husband Edward, she liked to drive fast, and she had driven an Army van in the Second World War. She was driving me along the main road from Montgomery to Newtown, near Castell Forwyn, where there is a bend in the road. The driver in front slowed down to 40 mph and my granny was complaining 'Come on man, you can go a bit faster!' I said to her, 'But Granny, I go that speed around that bend.' Her reply came back immediately: 'That's quite fast enough for you, dear!'

In July 1928, at an Oddfellows Montgomery District meeting, there was some potential political movement on pensions with promises from Neville Chamberlain who was now minister of health, but the Oddfellows were not seizing the moment. Sir Alfred Warren died the previous year so the senior team this year were now perhaps a little lacking in policy experience and influence. John was trying to chivvy them along, but it was an uphill battle:

> The district management committee reported that they had passed a resolution expressing the hope that the Grand Master and Board of Directors would submit a resolution on behalf of their society to the National Conference of Friendly Societies, in favour of the extension of the contributory pensions scheme to members of their Order who were not insured persons. A reply was received declining to forward the resolution... Bro. J.E. Tomley expressed regret at the decision of the Board...[18]

In September 1928, John was at the National Conference of Friendly Societies in Scarborough. The conference now represented over 8 million members. After the years of austerity, there was finally some good news with contributory pensions for some types of workers now starting to be paid as the final parts of the Pensions Act came into force. A new Unemployment Insurance Act had also been passed.[19]

In May 1929, John was at the Oddfellows' Annual Moveable Conference at Portsmouth. At the start of the meeting a list of women on the platform at the conference is given, including John's wife Edith, attending for the first time, now that more women were included.[20] Yet the next year, Edith had a serious accident. She may have been in the early stages of Huntington's disease.[21]

The idea of a national health service was discussed again at the National Conference of Friendly Societies in Blackpool in September 1930. The British Medical Association (BMA) had published a scheme to provide a general medical service for the nation – a national health service, but not a state-run one. At the same time, a cross-party group of MPs was looking at a separate scheme for a state medical service – getting closer to the idea of the national health service that was eventually created thanks to the pioneering work of John and others. [22]

Further roles

John continued to be appointed to other new roles through the 1920s. In 1925 he was appointed clerk to the justices of Montgomery at the same time as Sidney Pryce had left them to become mayor of the town. John was also appointed to the county-level Agricultural Wages Committee by the minister of agriculture, as well as becoming vice-chair of the Joint Committee for Wales and Monmouthshire which administered the pricing of more than two million prescriptions. This was the drugs pricing committee for National Insurance in Wales, an early equivalent to the National Institute for Health and Care Excellence (NICE) which recommends drugs today for the NHS, based on clinical effectiveness and price. As the Oddfellows Magazine put it: 'Another instance of the adage that it is the busy man who finds most time for public service.'[23]

The cost of these drugs was increasing and John became involved in investigating the reasons for this.[24] In October 1927, he explained how this work was progressing. He had been told that

> the amount of drugs used in Glamorgan was five times that used in Monmouth, and even in Merthyr Tydfil 100,000 prescriptions were made up annually. It stood to reason chemists could not supply unless they were paid in full, hence the clause in the new Government Bill would have to be watched and fought, because he foresaw the possibility of the insured person suffering. The remedy would be to battle for a separate Drug Fund for Wales.[25]

The committee met regularly. At another meeting in January 1930, the cost of special drugs was discussed, including insulin for people with diabetes, along with the inequality between payments made to panel doctors, which covered the full cost of special drugs, and those made to approved institutions, which were at a flat fee that did not cover the actual cost of more expensive drugs.

Another issue also occupied the meeting: 'It was reported that the Welsh Board of Health had approved of the consolidation of the salaries of the staff on the basis of a cost of living bonus of 70 per cent from October, 1929, to March, 1932, but there was no explanation as to the limitation of the period of approval…'[26] The second Labour-led government was now in power. Like the first, it was a minority government with a hung parliament, so it was hard for Labour to get their reforms through, and voters were disappointed. The economic situation meant that all public sector staff had to take pay cuts, so what sounds like a large 70 per cent 'cost of living bonus' in the meeting actually meant they had to only have 70 per cent of their previous salary in total: a cut of 30 per cent.

At the Association of Welsh Insurance Committees meeting two months later, the topics included two old chestnuts: doctors signing off excessive sickness certifications, and excessive prescribing. John was nominated to a Ministry of Health committee to tackle the latter.[27] Both happen because doctors are hard pressed for time and want to keep patients happy – exactly the same issues are faced by the NHS today.

The WNMA's work continues

Meanwhile John's work with the WNMA continued throughout the 1920s. A meeting in January 1925 at Aberystwyth heard about the role of light treatment after the WNMA's principal medical officer had seen it in action in Copenhagen. A new set-up in Cardiff had helped 'two chronic cases of lupus' and 'No one who had seen the light treatment in use could fail to be impressed with its importance in dealing with the tubercular diseases', so funding was sought for similar equipment in North Wales.

Mr D.W. Evans (the director of the North Wales Sanatorium), said Sir Robert Jones, one of the WNMA's consultant surgeons, had informed him that 'the sanatorium was the best equipped institution in the whole country. The only things lacking were light treatment appliances and a building to house them'. John asked what would be the approximate cost of the apparatus, and whether it would be available for ex-service men in North Wales. 'Mr Evans said the cost would be £400, and ex-service men would be eligible for treatment.'

The same meeting moved on to the issue of grants paid by the local authorities to the WNMA to fund its work. David Davies and others had given generously to set up the WNMA's hospitals and sanatoria. But when state funding was later found to do the same for England, the WNMA did not receive any extra state funding. The Finance Committee, which John was part of

> had decided to invite every County Council and County Borough Council to pass resolutions calling upon the Government to treat Wales in exactly the same way as English authorities had been treated, and calling upon members of Parliament to raise questions in Parliament and if necessary go as a deputation to the Chancellor of the Exchequer.

Mr Hopkin Morgan, from Neath, summed up feelings at the meeting when he said that 'Wales was being penalised because it had raised its capital expenditure by voluntary means'.

The WNMA was also seeing an increased number of patients, making extra funding even more crucial. 'The number of persons examined, treated, or recommended of the Association since the inception of the movement had reached the great total of 113,780, and of these 11,219 had received treatment in sanatoria and 22,390 in hospitals.'

While they had eradicated the waiting list for sanatoria, 157 people were still on the waiting list for hospital admissions, especially patients needing surgery. The director suggested that some patients recovering from surgery could be moved to sanatoria more quickly, to free up surgery beds. Small pavilions could be built at the sanatoria to house the extra patients. Yet this suggestion could not be put into action until further capital funding became available.[28]

In August 1925, for the first time a newspaper article featured John's TB statistics for all the Welsh counties, which he had been collecting for the national TB service run by the WNMA. This would become the most important work of his career. The article reported on the thirteenth annual meeting of the WNMA's board of governors, at Bangor. As usual, John used the numbers to reveal regional disparities:

> Mr J.E. Tomley, of Montgomery, called attention to statistics in the report showing the remarkable divergence between the Eastern and the Western counties of Wales in the matter of incidence of tuberculosis. Comparing each Western county with its neighbouring county for the year 1924, they found that while the deaths from tuberculosis in Caernarvonshire

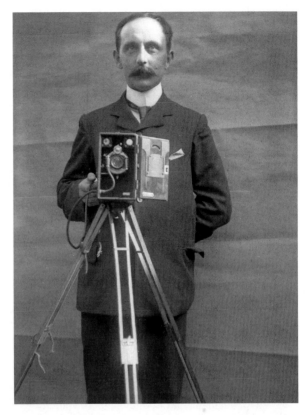

Right: John taking one of the first selfies in his home town of Montgomery, mid Wales, c.1905. (Photographer: John Tomley. *By permission of the Old Bell Museum, Montgomery*)

Below: Montgomery Town Hall, where John worked for Montgomery Town Council and Montgomeryshire County Council, c.1905. (Photographer: John Tomley. *From John Tomley's family papers*)

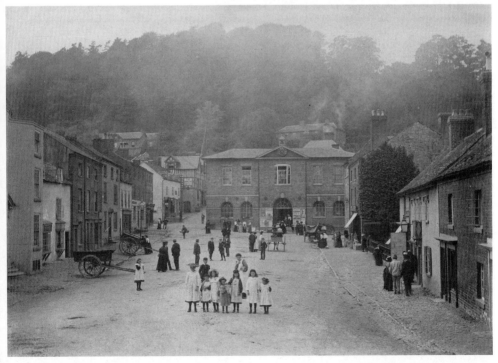

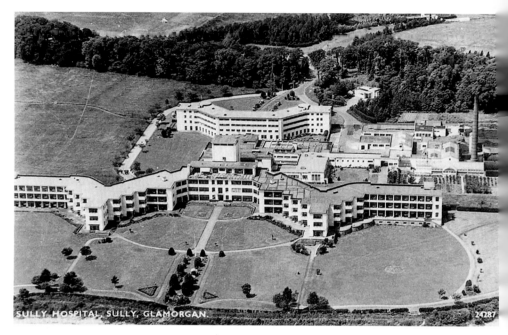

Above: Sully Hospital, the WNMA's flagship tuberculosis hospital, 1930s. (Photographer: Christopher Ware)

Below: Boys' trip, Montgomery, 1884. Based on family resemblances, this may have included John Tomley, age 10 (bottom row, far left), his father Robert, age 40 (directly above John), and Robert's council colleague Sidney Pryce, age 22 (top row, third from left). *From Sidney Pryce's family papers*

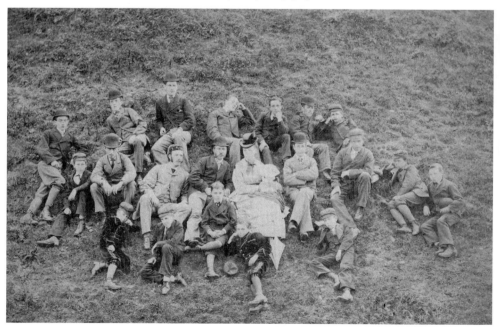

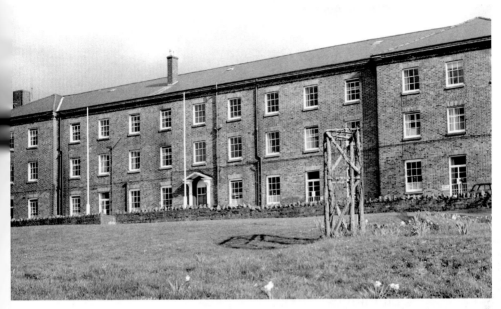

Forden Union Workhouse, c.1910. (*By permission of the Old Bell Museum, Montgomery*)

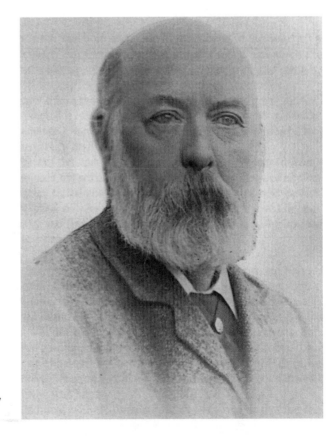

Dr Ray Snow, c.1900.
(*From Ray Snow's family papers*)

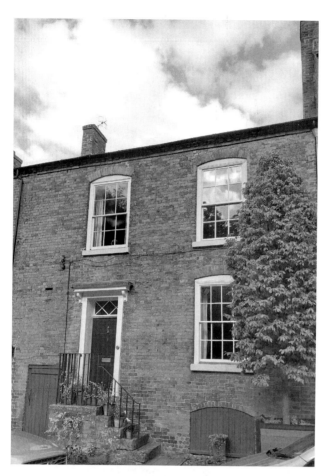

Left: Pryce, Tomley &
Pryce offices, 1 Arthur
Street, Montgomery.

Below: Sidney Pryce
& John Tomley in
Montgomery Cricket
Club, c.1890s. Top row,
second from left: Sidney
Pryce. Middle row,
second from right: John
Tomley. (Photographer
unknown. *From John
Tomley's family papers*)

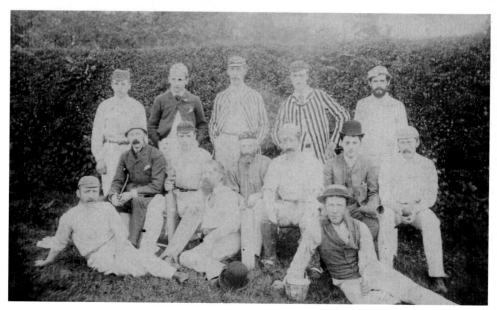

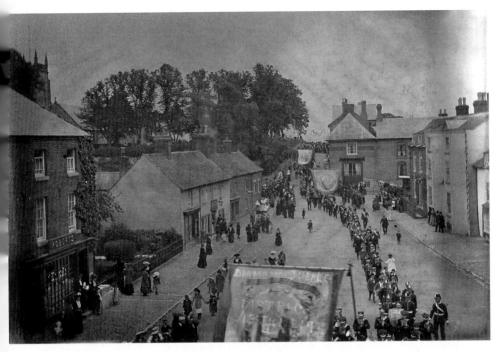

Above: Montgomery Oddfellows Golden Jubilee parade (Loyal Ark of Friendship Lodge), 23 June 1891. (*By permission of the Old Bell Museum, Montgomery*)

Below: Montgomeryshire Oddfellows branch banner, c. 1890s. (*By permission of the Old Bell Museum, Montgomery*)

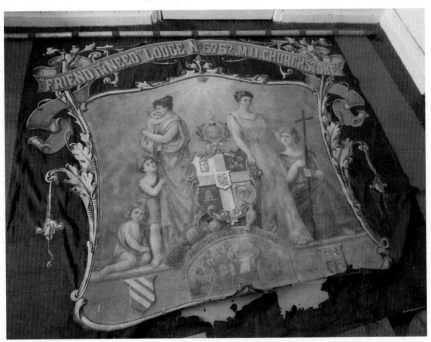

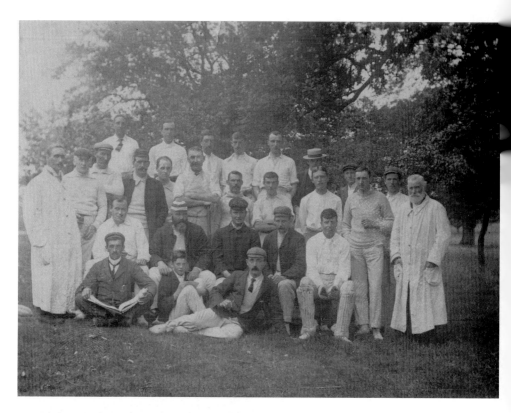

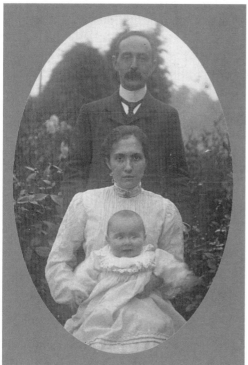

Above: John as captain of Montgomery Cricket Club, c.1905. Front row, seated on ground holding camera mechanism: John Tomley. Standing to far left: Sidney Pryce. (Photographer: John Tomley. *From John Tomley's family papers*)

Left: John, his wife Edith and one of their daughters, c.1905. (Photographer: John Tomley. *From John Tomley's family papers*)

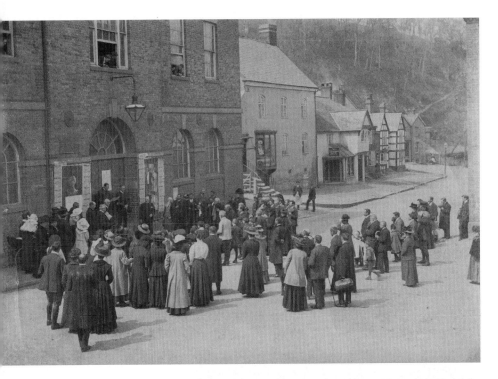

Above: Announcement of election of David Davies as MP, Montgomery Town Hall, 1906. Standing on step: left – Sidney Pryce announcing election result; right – David Davies. (Photographer: John Tomley. *From John Tomley's family papers*)

Right: Thomas Alders, the first person to claim the Old Age Pension in Montgomery, January 1909. (*By permission of the Old Bell Museum, Montgomery*)

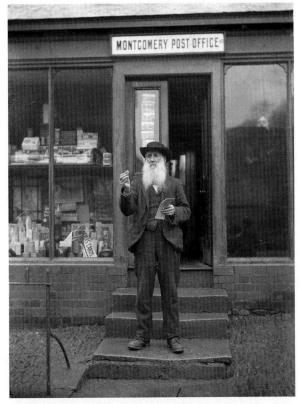

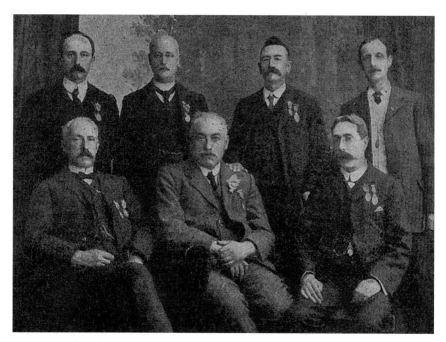

Above: John on the Oddfellows Investigation Committee, 1910 – top left. (*By permission of Manchester Unity of Oddfellows*)

Below: Invitation for Oddfellows Centenary Banquet, chaired by the Prince of Wales, 18 May 1910. (*From John Tomley's family papers*)

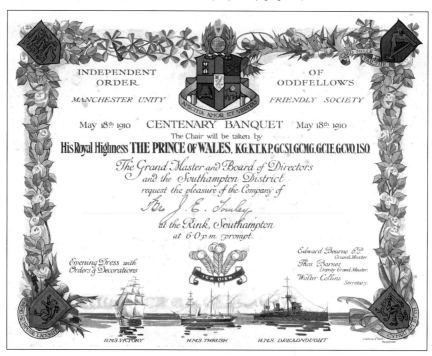

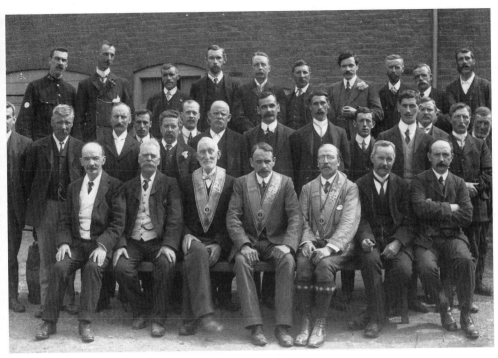

Above: Montgomeryshire Oddfellows branch, c.1914. John on bottom row, far right. (*By permission of the Old Bell Museum, Montgomery*)

Below and overleaf above: Land Girls in Montgomery during the First World War, hoeing turnips on Weston farm c.1915. John's wife Edith Tomley (top row, third from right); and daughters Esther (bottom row, far right) and Doris (bottom row, second from right). (*From John Tomley's family papers*)

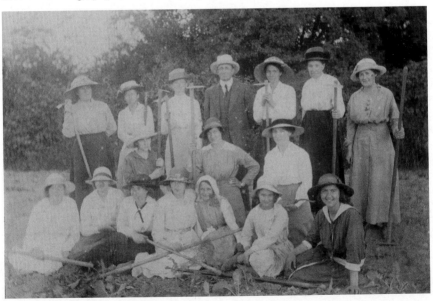

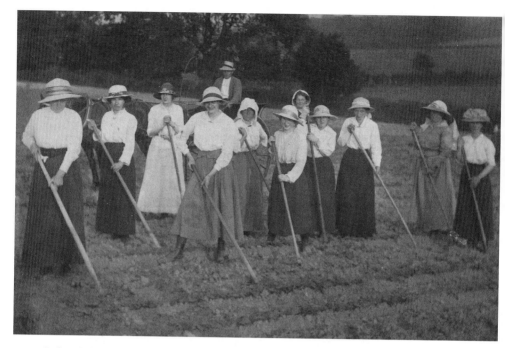

Below left: John, his wife Edith Tomley and their children (L to R) Esther, Edward and Doris c.1918. (*By permission of the Old Bell Museum, Montgomery*)

Below right: John at work c.1920. (*From John Tomley's family papers*)

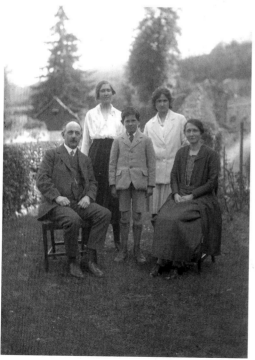

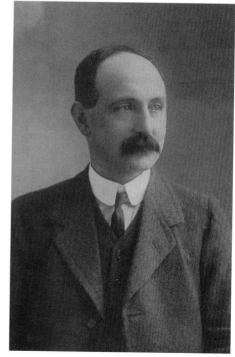

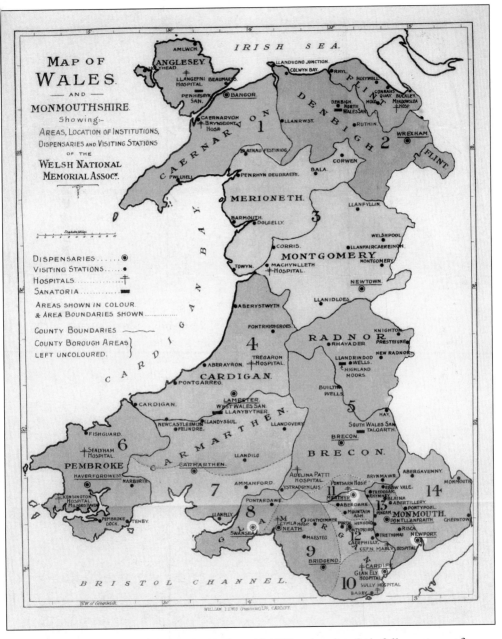

The WNMA's eventual services by the mid 1930s, showing their full coverage of Wales for TB services, including hospital, sanatorium and community services. (*By permission of the National Library of Wales*)

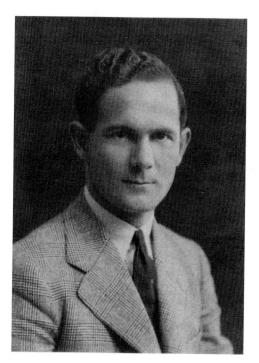

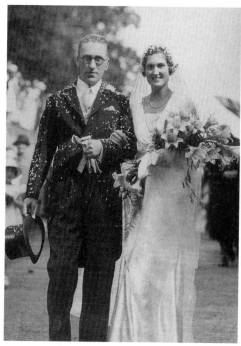

Above left: John's son Edward while working at his father's firm, c.1930s. (*From John Tomley's family papers*)

Above right: John's daughter Doris Tomley's marriage to Dr James (Jim) Stewart, 1933. (*From John Tomley's family papers*)

Below: John with his grandson David Stewart and daughter Doris, c.1939. (*From John Tomley's family papers*)

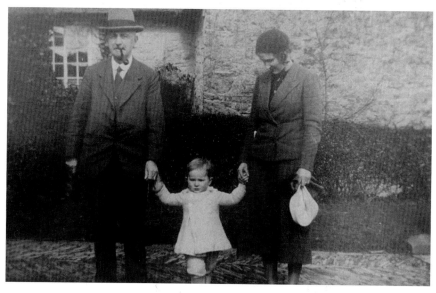

Montgomeryshire Insurance Committee.

Montgomery.

J.E.TOMLEY.
(Solicitor.)
CLERK.

Telephone P.O. N° 8

18th.December,1937.

Personal.

Dear Sir Kingsley,

I am delighted to learn that you are addressing a Public Meeting at Bangor in Caernarvonshire on January 19th.next because it is the sad fact that that County proves to have the highest rate of mortality from Tuberculosis amongst all the Counties of England,Wales and Scotland during the past seven years. This will be emphasised in the evidence which I shall have to give shortly before the Committee of Enquiry into the Anti-Tuberculosis arrangements in Wales which you have very wisely set up but it occurs to me that you may find it of some advantage to have an advance copy of the statistics in question. Their preparation has been quite a big job and, unfortunately the set required from your Department did not come to hand until some time after the Registrar General's statistical tables had been published. On the other hand the Scottish Registrar General,though it meant the preparation of some special schedules,very promptly complied with the request of our mutual friend Mr.Stanley Duff on behalf of the National Conference of Friendly Societies,of which I have to act as President.

Some other features in which I know you are keenly interested emerge from my tables e.g. the relative position of the sea-ports,especially on the North East Coast, with regard to Tuberculosis and the wonderful improvement shown during the last few years in this respect by the Metropolitan Boroughs. When I tell you that amongst all the 62 Counties of England and Wales seven Welsh Counties are bunched at the top of the list in respect of Tuberculosis mortality you will understand what a useful text for your address at Bangor my figures may supply. If they will be of service to you I will endeavour to have an advance proof supplied at once upon hearing from you.

Personal.   With all good wishes,
Sir Kingsley Wood,P.C.,M.P.   Yours sincerely,
Minister of Health,

Ministry of Health,
Whitehall, S.W.1.

Letter from John to Sir Kingsley Wood, Minister of Health. Ministry of Health files. (*By permission of the National Archives, Kew*)

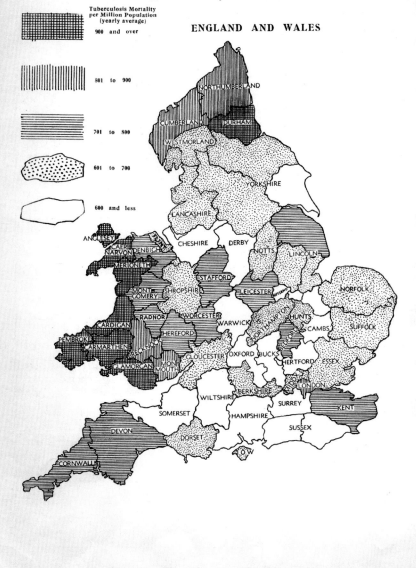

John's TB map of Wales, which opened the Welsh TB Inquiry. Ministry of Health files. (*By permission of the National Archives, Kew*)

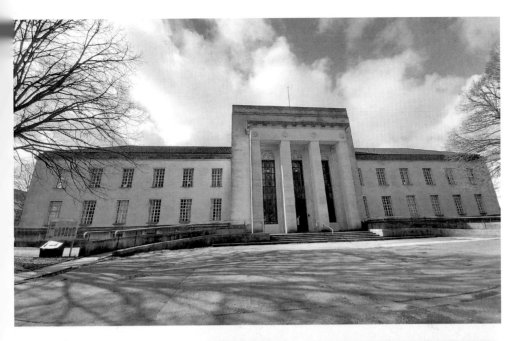

Above: Welsh Temple
of Peace and Health,
headquarters of the
WNMA.

Right: John as a Trustee
of Manchester Unity of
Oddfellows, wearing
his previous jewels and
other regalia. (*Oddfellows
Magazine*, 1934. *By
permission of Manchester
Unity of Oddfellows*)

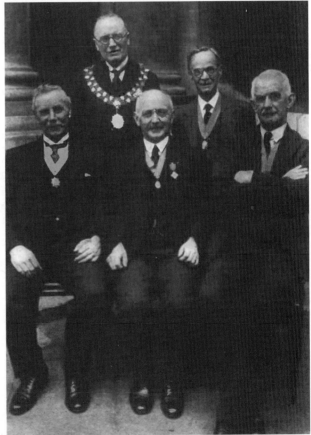

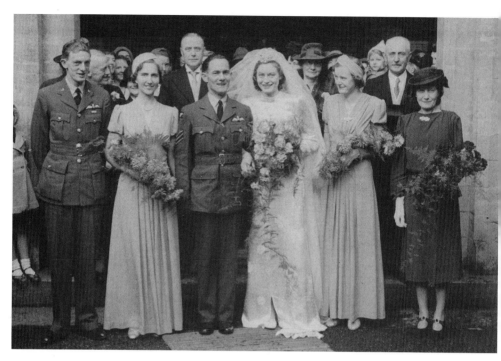

Above: John's son Edward Tomley's official marriage to Jose, 1942. Front row: John's daughter Esther (second from left), Edward and Jose (centre). Second row: John's wife Edith (second from right) and John (far right). (*From John Tomley's family papers*)

Below: John (second from left) with his daughter Doris (far left) and his nurse (second from right), c.1950. (*From John Tomley's family papers*)

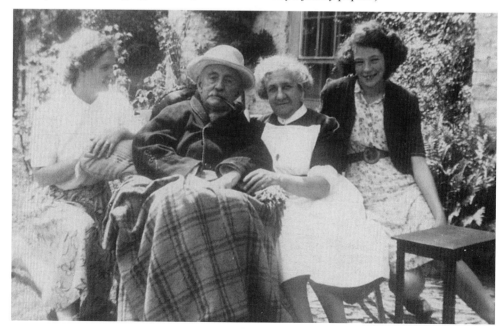

were at the rate of 1,705 per million, the Denbighshire figures were by 886. Merioneth, with 1,910 compared with the 910 of its Eastern neighbour Montgomery, and the 1,887 of Cardiganshire was also practically double the 946 of Radnor. The three counties which have had since 1911 the highest mortality from tuberculosis, Merioneth, Cardigan, and Carnarvon, had, at the last census, the smallest ration of children surviving under 15 to the thousand people... At the same time Cardigan and Merioneth had the highest percentage of widows, and the lowest proportion of married women. Again, in respect of mortality from tuberculosis, Cardigan, Carnarvon and Merioneth, headed the list in that order in 1911, and they still headed the list today...

And as usual, John also used his eloquence and the debating skills developed in his youth to bring home his point:

'Why is it', asked Mr Tomley, 'that in the parts of Wales where people live in the finest air, amongst the grandest natural surroundings God has given our land; where they mainly pursue healthy outdoor occupations, that this terrible scourge should be so rampant? Why is it that round our coasts, where those who live inland flock in their thousands to seek and to find invigoration, that so many of the residents weaken and die of tuberculosis? Is it not a problem capable of solution by our skilled medical advisers? Enough has been said to show that a sociological problem of first-rate importance is before us...'

John added that these rural counties suffered from young men migrating to industrial areas and getting ill, 'and many of these returned home stricken by the disease, and died from it, thereby increasing the incidence and the death rate'. He added how proud they could all be on the WNMA's efforts to tackle the disease and said to the applause of those present that the director of the WNMA 'Sir David Evans ought to have had his knighthood long ago'.[29]

By July 1926, however, they faced a crisis. Sir David Evans had died, which had hampered progress on all fronts, including the capital grants. Wales was still being penalised by the tuberculosis grants offered to England being withheld in Wales because of David Davies' past donations to fund land and buildings.

The WNMA was running out of capital, and David told another meeting that 'if Wales was to be treated as the English counties had been treated then at least another £50,000 was due from the Government' – but there was no sign this would be forthcoming: 'Preliminary negotiations with the Treasury had taken place during the past few weeks, but no definite promise of further assistance had yet been received.'

A rather controversial topic was discussed at the same WNMA meeting too. The WNMA was planning to do a research trial using a new treatment for TB, the Spahlinger method, resulting in 'a lively discussion'. Three of the WNMA's medical staff had visited Geneva to see Mr Spahlinger and his factory where he was trialling immunotherapy and a vaccine for TB. Some of the meeting delegates favoured trialling the treatment and giving the association 'fair play to pursue its investigations', whereas others felt it was a waste of money. Dr John Jones, on behalf of Merioneth County Council, strongly opposed the trial. 'It was cruel to go on with the inquiry at the expense of the ratepayers of Wales.' David Davies appealed to Dr Jones: 'It seemed to him that it was particularly the duty of the association to endeavour to get to the truth concerning the Spahlinger treatment.' David was on the side of history, of course – the Spahlinger treatment offered a successful vaccine.[30]

In November 1928, John gave a lengthy talk on 'The Finance Act, 1925 and the De-Rating Act' to Aberystwyth Chamber of Trade. The importance of this was that the lower average property values per resident in the county of Cardiganshire compared to Montgomeryshire meant Cardiganshire paid less rates per head. This meant less money, for example, for the local authority to pay to the WNMA for their TB services. However, the population's health needs and costs per head were likely to be the same in all areas.[31]

New senior roles

In early 1930, the *Oddfellows Magazine* reported that John 'has been appointed by the minister of health, Mr Arthur Greenwood, as a member of his advisory committee on the definition of drugs for the purposes of medical benefit' – and that 'Bro. Tomley has also been elected a Governor of the University College of Wales, Aberystwyth.'[32]

Today, that ministry of health committee's equivalent is the Medicines and Healthcare Products Regulatory Agency (MHRA), which regulates medicines, medical devices and blood components.

John's role on the Advisory Committee on the Definition of Drugs was not mentioned in the newspapers, so I only found it later on after looking in the Oddfellows archives. This is strange as this type of appointment was usually accompanied by a press release. I found the answer in the ministry of health files in The National Archives.

The committee, which had only been recently set up, had agreed at an initial meeting to include a representative of Wales. Instead of asking the Welsh Association of National Insurance Committees to nominate a representative, the overall UK body had been asked instead. They nominated someone from Wales who was offered the role. Then the Welsh Association of Insurance Committees heard about the role and sent their nominations in – for different people. This caused embarrassment as the first person had already been offered the role.

The Association of Welsh Insurance Committees were told that their nominee, their current president, was inappropriate as he also ran a pharmacy business so had a conflict of interest. John, as a past president and a member of another Ministry of Health committee looking at ratings valuations for railways, was suggested instead, but the Ministry refused. A lot of angry correspondence took place with the Welsh association accusing the UK association of going behind their backs. Finally, the situation was resolved when the person who had been offered the role stepped down due to becoming an MP – and possibly due to talks that had happened with them behind the scenes. The role was quickly offered to John instead. The whole thing was so sensitive and embarrassing that a Ministry of Health memo shows civil servants actively chose not to do a press release for John's appointment, for fear of inflaming people's opinions again.

So now John was on another Ministry of Health committee – but was it useful? In some ways these committees were quite boring and more of a talking shop than a place to get things done.

Even before John joined the Advisory Committee on the Definition of Drugs, the Ministry of Health correspondence files show the doctor chairing the committee complaining to the senior civil servant who appointed him:

> I must get out of that Definition of Drugs Committee. It has become a nightmare... All we have done at the last two or three meetings, which is almost nothing, might have been done far better, it seems to me, in five minutes by yourself. How am I to get out of it?

The reply came back from the civil servant, after a calming introduction about some excellent claret wine: 'don't resign', noting that 'of course they include some expert conversationalists'. It worked – the doctor stayed on.

The first task of the committee was to decide which products were drugs, i.e., medicines which should be dispensed by pharmacists and paid for by health insurance, and which were not. You might say this was easy, yet it had been prompted by a recent medical breakthrough – vitamin supplements. The government did not want to commit to buying vitamin supplements for the whole population because it would be unaffordable, yet a lot of people had vitamin deficiencies so supplements were a medical necessity. So they became a class called 'Sometimes a medicine' which meant it depended on the circumstances.

Other supplements, from Oxo to Eno's Fruit Salt, were also looked at by the committee. Where the ingredients were published by the manufacturer and doctors agreed there was a medical benefit for people lacking in certain nutrients, they joined the class of 'Sometimes a medicine' too. Yet for other supplements where the manufacturer published no ingredients list, the committee said that doctors should no longer use the products and they would not be paid for by health insurance. When the list was published, shortly before John joined the committee, manufacturers and doctors were up in arms. In a number of cases, useful items had been excluded which were vital to people's health. The ingredients of many items were not publicly available yet were shown in medical journals read by doctors, so were safe to use. Several manufacturers threatened to sue. A revised list was quickly rushed out. Following the embarrassment, some 'disciplinary action' is referred to in the committee minutes, and we are told at the next meeting that the female civil servant who was administering the committee is no longer working in the role.

John joined after the list with errors was published, so most committee meetings after this were taken up with the legal proceedings. The committee did not last much longer before being disbanded. A number of years later, it was set up again in its modern incarnation, which eventually became the MHRA.

The useful part of the role was that John had been officially appointed to this committee by the minister of health, although the minister himself did not necessarily attend the committee meetings. What it did mean was that John was now able to write directly to the minister via letters marked 'personal' – as the protocol was that the minister's staff did not open these letters. John was also able to put letters directly in the hands of the minister when they met at events. In this way, he was able to manage to get around the minister's gatekeepers, senior civil servants who were keen to maintain the status quo. Unfortunate ideas such as setting up a national health service run by the government were clearly unthinkable to them, as it would not only involve a lot of work for these senior staff, but also, in contrast to people like John and David Davies, they had no qualifications or experience in running a health service directly, so might lose their jobs.

I was fascinated to find several bulging Ministry of Health files in The National Archives featuring John. As well as the two committees, there were also files of John's personal correspondence with the ministers over the years, and John's crucial evidence for the TB inquiry which would be a major milestone on the road to the NHS, as we will see.

Surprisingly, the other appointment of John's mentioned at the same time, as a governor of Aberystwyth University, turned out to be very useful for networking with ministers of health too. As well as David Davies as president, another governor was Nye Bevan MP, the future minister of health. The university's students had a high rate of TB, so the governors would have discussed health services together.

A Wireless Community

Despite all this committee activity, John still found time to campaign for practical local health service improvements in his role as a local health commissioner. In 1930, he contributed his third article to David Davies' *Welsh Outlook* magazine, 'A Wireless Community', bemoaning 'One hundred square miles of country-side without a single telephone!' at the eastern end of Montgomeryshire where it converged with the counties of Cardigan and Merioneth. In a fabulously modern vision, John suggests the invention of wireless phones, i.e. mobile phones, to call doctors in an emergency in rural areas. This did of course happen in the end, yet it took another 50 years until my childhood in the 1980s.

> It seems ludicrous, if it were not so pathetic, that the dweller on our hill-sides can by the flick of a switch bring into his home the music of a jazz band, but cannot by any wireless action or by any human means, until perhaps too late, secure medical aid for a sufferer in agony.
>
> The needs of these rural communities are well illustrated by the fact that in an area on the western side of Co. Montgomery covering 420 square miles, there is no doctor. In the whole of this territory there are only fifteen telephone call offices. Such a state of things would not be tolerated in Norway or Sweden. Why should our patient sufferers be compelled to endure it here?[33]

Chapter 5

'An Inquiry in My Own Way'
1931–1937

John continued his main paid work as a local health commissioner throughout the 1930s. Increasingly, his work started overlapping with his voluntary work for the friendly societies and on the board of the WNMA, the Welsh national TB service.

John remained closely involved with the Association of Welsh Insurance Committees, representing local health commissioners across Wales. He was on their executive committee, after his earlier stint as president. At committee meetings, he continued to raise the issues of the incidence of tuberculosis, as well as the cost of drugs. Prevention would be better than cure, then fewer drugs would be needed, as there would be fewer patients.[1]

Meanwhile, as a local health commissioner in Montgomeryshire, John set up an experimental national health service local pilot scheme, treating both insured and uninsured members of friendly societies. In 1932, John invited two senior national health leaders to an event in Montgomeryshire to hear about his new pilot: John Rowland, chairman of the Welsh Board of Health, and the Oddfellows' grand master, Bro. T.R. Morgan. John would have been hoping for approval from these visitors with national influence, so that he might be able to replicate the pilot elsewhere and roll it out nationally.

John met the visitors with his boss, Major J. Burdon-Evans, JP, vice-chairman of the county council and chairman of the National Health Insurance Committee for Montgomeryshire, the local health commissioning body, where John was clerk.

John explained, as reported in the *Oddfellows Magazine*:

> The happiest relations existed between the Insurance Committee and the district, and also between the medical men of county. In Montgomeryshire there was a unique arrangement with the medical men of the county. It was due to the Insurance Committee and Major Burdon-Evans that arrangements were made with all the medical men

in the county, without exception, to undertake to attend professionally all the members of friendly societies, adults and juveniles, even if they were not insured members.

Major Burdon-Evans then went on to say that the Welsh Board of Health 'had done well, but he thought they might have done even better if they had not been so closely controlled by Whitehall'. Later we find out the Welsh Board of Health staff were based in London and not in Wales, the area they were meant to be looking after.

John Rowland seems to have felt a bit put on the spot by this, retorting defensively: 'Whatever our shortcomings we are endeavouring to give of our best for the services of Wales in health matters...' Remember this for later – John Rowland was an important gatekeeper to the minister of health and John had offended him. And there wasn't just this suggestion of an amalgamated medical service, but all those years John had spent fighting the Welsh Health Insurance Commissioners too – John Rowland was one of them and had a long memory, as we shall see later.[2]

On the opposite page of the *Oddfellows Magazine*, there was an article about subsidized spa treatment now being offered for National Health insured members with rheumatism and similar diseases. This had been debated before at the National Conference of Friendly Societies, but with no knowledge of its clinical effectiveness it had been difficult to make any decision about recommendation of treatment or funding. Now the new Ministry of Health had brought in the ideas of clinical effectiveness and financial business cases, and had collected the required information. It was calculated that rheumatic diseases were costing the country £17 million a year when wages and other losses were taken into account as well as leading to 'incalculable pain and suffering' and 'a vast amount of unhappiness'.

John was still involved in similar Ministry of Health work in relation to prescription medicines, so this article gives us some insight into his work. He also used this business case approach to good effect in a later medical journal article about TB and used his T.B. death statistics to enquire into clinical effectiveness of different approaches. This meant that his arguments stood a much better chance of being adopted by the Ministry of Health.

Still rising among the Oddfellows

During the early 1930s, John continued his voluntary work as a trustee of the Oddfellows. In May 1931, at the Oddfellows' annual conference in

Scarborough, the Investigation Committee chaired by John reported that they had seen the highest ever number of grant applications to the distress fund in the past quarter century since he had joined the committee, showing the severe levels of hardship being faced across the country due to the economic circumstances.

It sounds like the conference had become a much more sociable occasion with dancing and some new technology in the form of a gramophone record of the Oddfellows' song, 'the audience taking up the choruses as the record was played. The… record was one of the Board's propaganda efforts. Brother Watcyn Watcyn, the famous Queen's Hall singer, sang the Oddfellows' song, and was also a member of the quartet which sang the opening ode.'[3] While this may sound frivolous, it was actually for a very good purpose – to attract new young members to the Oddfellows so that they would be protected in times of sickness and unemployment.

In September 1931, John was at the National Conference of Friendly Societies in Margate, where the president, Bro. Herbert White, spoke of 'the conditions of national storm and stress which engage our minds at this time'. While the value of friendly societies' investments had fortunately stayed stable, Britain had to come off the gold standard that year due to the economic depression. This meant each pound was shrinking in purchasing value and so people were less able to cover their living costs from their friendly society benefits. 'Failure to maintain that value means immediate penury and misery in the homes of the sick, the sorrowing, and the aged,' warned White.

John spoke about the issue of private patients, which remains a controversial issue in the NHS today. The BMA had lobbied the minister of health to add a clause to allow insured patients to be treated privately by a second doctor, as long as it was not their appointed panel doctor who was already paid for through their health insurance. It was probably a sweetener to the doctors, who had agreed to reduce the huge fees they were getting. 'The second doctor would be subject to no regulation whatever as to treatment and certificates,' John told the conference. Bro. Meadmore recommended that 'panel patients should be warned by their friendly society against being manoeuvred into a position in which they would be made to pay as private patients'.[4]

In May 1932, John was at the Oddfellows' Annual Moveable Conference in Guernsey, chairing the Investigation Committee as usual. He had been elected 25 times for the committee, a record for the Oddfellows. It was decided to hold the next conference in London, as John had proposed a year earlier, 'seeing as it was to be a conference of an unusual character'.

The Oddfellows were hoping for 'such publicity for the Manchester Unity as they had never yet had', and 'for the attendance at that Conference of such important personages as would give them an overwhelming standing.'[5] John was certainly planning something.

In September, at the National Conference of Friendly Societies in Leicester, John was elected to the Standing Orders Committee – part of the executive. The keynote speaker at the conference was Mr Ernest Brown, M.P., Parliamentary Secretary to the Ministry of Health, who spoke about the high rate of women dying in childbirth.

Again, delegates discussed a full national health service, 'with the extension and co-ordination of existing medical services, for the provision of a more complete medical service for insured persons and the extension thereof to their dependents'.[6]

A year on, in 1933, John became a member of the executive committee, and the president raised a national health service again, but only for insured people, not reaching the people who most needed it who were unemployed, pregnant or had disabilities. John was probably starting to think that he could do better himself if he was the president...[7]

Elected to the Oddfellows board

The next year, in January 1934, the Oddfellows Montgomeryshire District voted for John to be nominated as a Director of the Oddfellows nationally. John explained he would have to give up his Investigation Committee nomination as people were only allowed one or the other.[8] A vote took place in May and he was duly elected to the board, a separate role from being a trustee:

> Bro. Director Tomley said it... was a great pleasure to him to think that they had honoured one who came from a little country of which very little had been heard that week – that was the principality of Wales. It was not often that a member of the Celtic race was honoured with a seat on the Board... He trusted that he would be endowed with health and strength to serve them loyally and well.

In the coming year, John would attend numerous Oddfellows events, speaking or presenting 'Jewels', the Oddfellows' special ribbon medals, and sometimes accompanied by Edith. His suggestion of holding the

Oddfellows' annual conference in London to attract senior political figures to attend had proved prescient. He and the other directors had managed a fantastic policy and influence coup. Not just a health minister, but a prime minister: former Tory prime minister Stanley Baldwin, who would be re-elected the following year, spoke at the conference, which was held in the Royal Albert Hall. The *Oddfellows Magazine* as ever was on hand:

> Mr Baldwin [has]... a personal knowledge of the good work done in the lives of working men by the friendly societies.... In a world where so many things are rocking to ruin we have escaped revolutions and dictatorships because we know the principles of a democracy which our people will never let go.
>
> This led Mr Baldwin to the conclusion that the day will never come when the work of our friendly societies will no more be necessary... Nothing more helpful and appropriate has been heard at any of our annual conferences than the words of one who was an active Oddfellow before he became a statesman and Prime Minister.[9]

In October 1934, John was invited to a dinner with the Prince of Wales again – a different man, of course, this time the future King Edward VIII – and this time he was able to attend. The Foresters' Centenary Dinner took place at the Guildhall. 'I look on this as a very important occasion,' declared the prince. 'Friendly societies such as yours have played a leading part in our social history. They are held in very high esteem.'[10]

Later that month, John was the keynote speaker at the Oddfellows' South Wales and Monmouthshire conference about the high incidence of illness in South Wales.

> In his recent report Sir George Newman, Chief Medical Officer of the Ministry of Health, referred to 10 Welsh counties as being among the 14 counties in England and Wales responsible for high maternal mortality rates, and also to the fact that in Glamorgan last year practically 1,000,000 prescriptions were issued by doctors to insured persons. It was computed that 435 prescriptions were issued to every 100 insured persons in the area. Swansea had the distinction of consuming the greatest amount of medicine in the whole of Wales. These prescription forms, if placed end to end, would reach from Swansea to Cardiff and back again.[11]

A new WNMA hospital

John's work with WNMA continued to move forward through the early 1930s. In November 1931, the WNMA was planning a new hospital in Sully in South Wales. This was a beautiful new state of the art hospital, with an award-winning art deco design which is now Grade II listed, facing south towards the Bristol Channel. It was perfect for TB patients to relax and recover on balconies attached to their wards, over multiple floors. The estimated cost was £150,000. Yet public sector staff were being asked to take pay cuts to help the government during the economic crisis.

The president at the WNMA's event detailing the plans was John's old ally David Davies, who was 'heartily congratulated... on his election as honorary Freeman of the City of Cardiff'. The *Western Mail* report on the proposals indicates that as usual John Tomley was a key player:

> Thanks were expressed to Mr J.E. Tomley (Montgomery) for his services in compiling statistics and charts showing the incidence of tuberculosis throughout Wales. These data were referred to the medical committee for inquiry...
>
> The President said it was important to try to ascertain the causes of such a high mortality from tuberculosis in certain districts when other districts were comparatively immune, and Mr Tomley's investigations and data would be of great assistance in the matter.

The Ministry of Health had agreed the hospital at Sully 'was required on urgent grounds of public health and the council were recommended to proceed with the scheme'. Meanwhile, on the cost-cutting theme:

> The finance committee expressed appreciation of the willingness of the medical, nursing and administrative staffs to make a voluntary contribution to meet the present financial situation, and the offer was accepted by the council on the following lines: An abatement of 10 per cent on salaries of £1,000 and over; 7 ½ per cent on salaries between £750 and £1,000; and the N.A.L.G.O. scale of reduction on all salaries between £156 and £750...[12]

This is the last time the press mention 'Mr' David Davies. In 1929 he had stood down as an MP at the general election, and was succeeded by

Clement Davies as MP for Montgomeryshire. In 1932, thanks mainly to his work setting up the WNMA's TB service in Wales, the first national health service, David was made Lord Davies of Llandinam for services to health.

In July 1933, there was a new development, with John attending a conference in Cardiff run by the National Association for the Prevention of Tuberculosis, which changed its focus over time and still exists today as the Stroke Association. Once again John was on hand with the data:

> Mr J.E. Tomley, clerk to the Montgomeryshire Insurance Committee, spoke of the incidence of tuberculosis in relation to the Welsh-speaking people... The reasons for this coincidence of language and mortality, he said, might be argued interminably in answer to such questions as whether Welsh people are content to remain domiciled in primitive and unhealthy surroundings; whether they are clannish in their inter-marriages; whether they have a national characteristic of fatalism, and will not seek or accept specialised treatment for the disease, or whether the whole secret is some mysterious national physical weakness which makes native Welsh people more susceptible and prone to this 'white plague'.

John, of course, was perfectly aware of the link between housing and disease, and was setting up the question of race, which many people still believed to be a cause of TB, in order for the doctors to come in and explain why issues with Welsh people as a race were no longer thought to be the cause.

Dr R.J. Peters, senior assistant medical officer of health for Glasgow, in a paper about TB and housing was there to clearly state that 'There is a marked correlation between mortality rates from these [respiratory] diseases and a poor standard of housing.' He, too, was an advocate of good data:

> In houses of one apartment [one room], the incidence of pulmonary tuberculosis was 1.52 per 1,000, in two-apartment houses, the rate was practically the same, but in four-apartment houses it had fallen to 1.06. A correction for differences in age and sex distribution [shows] the net proportional result is that in houses of four and more apartments the incidence of pulmonary tuberculosis is less than two-thirds of that in one-apartment houses.'[13]

National Conference executive committee

In September 1934, John was at the National Conference of Friendly Societies at Torquay, as a member of the executive committee for the past year, and had been working on a report on TB. The president this year, Bro. T.G. Graham from the Oddfellows, was much more forward thinking than his predecessor, and opened up the field for John to champion health prevention as being a key aim of the national friendly society movement. Graham told the conference:

> At the birth of National Health Insurance its primary purpose as it grew up and developed was to preserve health and incidentally to contribute to the alleviation of sickness. How much have we done by the aid of National Health to preserve the health of the nation? ...
>
> To prevent sickness is better constructive work than to cure it. Have we not made the mistake of accepting sickness as an inescapable fact rather than going upon the more helpful line of preventing it?... For over 20 years we have been engaged in fights, sometimes against the Ministry, more frequently against the legislation of Parliament, and the ring in which those fights have been waged has always been the money ring.
>
> I am indebted to Bro. J.E. Tomley for a report prepared in relation to the causes of the continued high death-rate from tuberculosis in certain parts of North Wales.... I am indebted to Bro. Tomley for giving me one of the most uncomfortable half-days of my life in reading that book – a tragic epitome of the sacrifice of commonplace lives in conditions which should be a challenge to the humanitarianism of every Friendly Society man in this country.

The president continued with a list of the friendly societies' achievements but tempered by a stern call for more to be done, again with the focus on prevention:

> We have lost great opportunities in having concerned ourselves as to the administration of benefits rather than to lay hold of the social side of these things which would have carried us back to causes... We have had, and we have to-day, plenty of material for the creation of a great Health force in our national life. Let us keep our minds centred on our

material resources and the way in which we could use them
for the building up of better homes and a healthier Britain.[14]

Next in the conference there was a speech by Isaac Foot, a Liberal MP
whose then 20-year-old son Michael would later lead the Labour Party.
'Big things depended on the friendly societies for, after all, civilization was
a precarious thing, and it was their privilege to extend it,' he said. Michael
had just graduated from Oxford University and had got a job as a shipping
clerk in Birkenhead, where he would be hugely influenced by the poverty
and unemployment he saw in Liverpool at that time, before working with
Nye Bevan and becoming a Labour MP himself in 1945, helping with the
founding of the NHS and welfare state.

You might have wondered how John managed to maintain his law career
with so many different activities going on, and so many committees he was
on. Helpfully, in January 1933, his son Edward had passed his Law Society
final examination and qualified as a solicitor. Aged 23, young and handsome,
Edward was cheeky and still a little wild, more interested in fast cars and
girls than John would have liked. Yet Edward was able to take responsibility
at work, and John could now start to leave Edward looking after his business
more. This meant John now had the opportunity to play a national leadership
role in the friendly societies' movement, a role which he had been offered yet
had kept turning down for so long while his family were growing up.[15]

Consultative Council on National Health Insurance

On 13 December 1934, Hansard, the parliamentary record, reported that
John had been appointed to the government's Consultative Council on
National Health Insurance (Approved Societies Work) with effect from 1
October 1934, to represent the Oddfellows. This was part of the Ministry
of Health. The council was chaired by a Druid – or, rather, Mr J.W. Shaw
of the Order of Druids Friendly Society. Although it is amusing to imagine
that the twentieth-century government still used to consult the Druids, as
in Roman times, of course this form of modern Druidry (distinct from the
neopagan type) was another friendly society movement.

Many years earlier, John had been nominated for this committee but had
been left off the list, probably due to having annoyed the Welsh Insurance
Commissioners too much when he stood up to them about the issues in the
National Health Insurance Act. Now someone had finally decided it was
John's turn.

The minutes are held in the Ministry of Health papers in The National Archives. For John's first meeting in May 1935, there were only two items on the agenda. First, a statement by the minister of health with regard to new health and pensions legislation, to be followed by a discussion on the effect of unemployment on (a) duration of insurance and (b) arrears of contributions. Second, discussion of memoranda dealing with certain proposed amendments of the National Health Insurance Act mainly of an administrative character.

This agenda and the meeting papers and minutes in the same file proved illuminating. The Ministry of Health was clearly not overly keen on consultation with the friendly societies. The committee only met once per year. The meeting invitations were only sent out by post a few weeks in advance. Allowing for delivery time, many of the attendees would only have a couple of weeks' notice. This was too little for senior people running health services. Therefore, each meeting file contains a lot of letters of apology.

The first year, John managed to get to the meeting on 10 May 1935. The minister of health was present – Sir Hilton Young MP, who would within days be replaced by Sir Kingsley Wood MP, both Conservatives.

The minutes do not record John speaking at the meeting. This may well have been because it was his first meeting and he wanted to get the lie of the land. Alternatively, he might have already seen that the real solutions to poverty and health at this time of extremely high unemployment lay elsewhere and not in fiddling around the edges with the current legislation. Megan Lloyd George, MP for Anglesey, was also attending the same meetings. As John knew her father, the former prime minister, through David Davies, she was to prove to be a useful parliamentary connection.

The next year, so many people couldn't attend the meeting planned for June 1936 that it was rescheduled to December. This time, the main topic being discussed was voluntary pensions insurance for 'black-coated workers', an extension of the National Insurance scheme to more industries. This time, the minister of health was not there. This time, John was able to get a word in edgeways in the discussions, mentioning the difficulty in assessing incomes in agricultural districts and the higher level of mileage fees in rural areas.

The next year, 1937, John had to send his apologies to the meeting due to a clash with the first meeting of the newly elected Montgomeryshire County Council, where John was the county returning officer. Then that was that – he dropped off the lists of attendees with no explanation in the minutes. Possibly everyone was on a three-year term so his term expired.

John no doubt realized there were better ways to spend his time to get real social change than to be on this committee. Yet the main advantage to John of being on the Ministry of Health committees was for a different purpose – to get direct contact with the minister of health to seek influence to achieve social policy change.

TB statistics

1935 was to prove a momentous year for John's TB statistics work. By the end of the year, he had managed to get an important journal paper published.

In March, John persuaded Clement Davies, the MP for Montgomeryshire, to take up the cause of the high TB rates in Wales in Parliament for the first time. An article John wrote for the *Oddfellows Magazine*, 'The scourge of Wales: high rate of mortality from tuberculosis', subtitled 'How England and Scotland lead', shortly afterwards explains the outcome. In the debate in the House of Commons, Clement Davies called for an inquiry 'so that we may have the causes ascertained and then do our best to remove them', supported by other Welsh MPs. The government representative Geoffrey Shakespeare MP, parliamentary secretary for the Ministry of Health, had said 'It is true that the figures in Wales are higher than those in England, but over the last decade there has been a noticeable fall'. This wasn't enough for John, who wrote:

> It was not revealed in the reply on behalf of the Ministry of Health that, while the death rate in Wales decreased from 1,179 to 986 between 1923 and 1933, the corresponding decrease for England and Wales was from 1,062 to 824. The Annual Report for 1933 of the Council of the National Association for the Prevention of Tuberculosis states: 'Within twenty years the mortality in England from all forms of tuberculosis has fallen approximately 41 per cent. In Scotland the decline in mortality has been 50 per cent.' In Wales the decrease between 1913 and 1933 has been only 22 per cent... In Brecon there were only seven fewer deaths in 1933 than in 1911. The population was 2,000 less. These, and scores of other terrible facts are the challenge to action.[16]

In a later *Oddfellows Magazine*, John explained his thinking up to this point and the work he carried out in 1935 writing a booklet with TB mortality statistics. He referenced an earlier WNMA report detailing the 'dismal housing conditions, lack of sanitary facilities, defective sewerage arrangements, tainted water supply, unsatisfactory milk supply and unsuitable dietary in one particular area of North Wales' – but that the government was complacent in its responses. John wrote of what he called 'An inquiry... in my own way':

> That did not take matters much further so, with the cordial encouragement of the members of the Welsh Board of Health and the whole-hearted co-operation of the principal officers of the Welsh National Memorial Association, I set about an inquiry in that year (1935) in my own way. This took the form of an 'Analysis of Tuberculosis Mortality in Wales, 1930-33.' In a booklet of 30 quarto pages I showed the actual areas in Wales where the incidence of T.B. mortality remained abnormally high, tracing them out, not merely as counties, but right down to the smaller administrative areas in each county.[17]

Later in the year John also presented more statistics to the WNMA, including an analysis of Wales's university towns of Aberystwyth, Bangor and Cardiff having unexpectedly high rates of TB, including 'a relatively large number of teachers falling victims' – an issue familiar again from the recent coronavirus pandemic. John supported 'Dr Emrys Jones's recommendation that only healthy students be admitted to State-aided schemes in our higher education centres'.[18]

Ministry of Health correspondence

Since the early 1930s, John had made sure to make the most of his first senior Ministry of Health role, as a member of the Advisory Committee on the Definition of Drugs, and his later role on the Consultative Council on National Health Insurance. While the committee meetings themselves were fairly pointless, they gave John good access to the minister of health.

The Ministry of Health correspondence files in The National Archives show that in 1935, John sent his report, 'Analysis of Tuberculosis Mortality in Wales, 1930-33' to the minister of health, backed up by questions asked by Clem Davies MP. A Ministry of Health staff member, Dr MacNalty, asked another doctor, Dr Chapman, to look at John's statistics and see whether they needed looking into further. The reply that comes back in the Ministry of

Health files in July 1935 is a masterfully worded example of shooting the messenger – basically saying that the subject should be analysed in a different way. In their experience, where young adult death rates are high the death rate could only be expected to decline slowly, which is why Wales was behind England, so TB mortality in Wales should not be looked into further. Also some areas of Wales had a small population so were statistically insignificant. In fact, we later see that the real issue was poverty – so there was something that could be done. Chapman's reply declared:

> I have read Mr Tomley's report 'An Analysis of Tuberculosis Mortality in Wales', but I do not find that it gets to the root of the matter... It is our inevitable experience that where 'young adult' mortality is relatively high the death rate at all ages declines but slowly. Wales conforms to this experience.
>
> I should have thought, therefore, that Mr Tomley should have worked the subject from this angle and discussed what can be done to improve matters. Instead there are only occasional and somewhat incidental references to adult mortality... On the whole I find little of value in the report and I fear it is not likely to be helpful.[19]

It seemed that John had come to a dead end.

Yet John's policy magic was still working. In the meantime, while the Ministry of Health were dismissing his work, he had a lucky breakthrough elsewhere, with academics at the Royal Sanitary Institute. This turned out to be a career-defining moment.

Tuberculosis and National Health Insurance journal paper

Also in 1935, John had to cover for Bro. Bertram, the president of the National Conference of Friendly Societies, who was ill. John took his place as a speaker at the Royal Sanitary Institute Congress at Bournemouth, and wrote an accompanying paper.[20] Now here was a chance for John to make his mark. Yet this opportunity had come about entirely by accident, and at very short notice. Could he make it work? Could he move fast enough to make use of this opportunity? John dropped everything and got down to work straight away.

The end result was that John took his greatest personal step towards the creation of the modern NHS, when he made the first fully costed business case for a universal national health service covering everyone in the UK, funded by universal national health insurance. He made the point that tuberculosis could not be fully dealt with unless and until everyone in the country was treated, as otherwise the untreated people keep reinfecting others. This meant not just all workers, but also their wives, children and older people. Also, all causes of tuberculosis needed to be dealt with, including overcrowded homes with poor sanitation.

John's ground-breaking journal article was published in a leading national public health journal, the *Journal of the Royal Sanitary Institute* (now *Perspectives in Public Health*), in April 1935.

Despite the rush job with preparing the paper, John was clearly successful, as his idea of a national health service was picked up by the BMA by the time he became the president of the National Conference of Friendly Societies himself just three years later.

So, what was the main point of this article? It appears to be mainly about setting out the statistics for health insurance and sickness benefits, with a particular focus on TB given his knowledge of this area, in the context of the huge cost to society of people being ill. And he advocates gathering data wherever possible:

> The preparation of an analysis of the records of the whole of the Approved Societies of the country, setting out the proportion of these millions of weeks of sickness which was due to each of the multitude of ills which beset us would be an enormous task; but there are some features of the morbidity experience of the societies which it would be to the advantage of their members and the general public to collate and make known.

And again, reminds the reader of the importance of preventative measures:

> There is amongst all these administrative bodies which exist for beneficent purposes in connection with our communal life and well-being a common interest not merely to comfort and relieve the distress and suffering of the afflicted, but to serve the nation by tracing and stamping out any preventable causes of the spread of the disease which may be found to exist.

As we might expect, he is particularly eloquent on TB:

> The yearly toll of fatal road accidents forms a constant subject of agitation in the press, but the deaths from tuberculosis

are more than five times as many – yet we have no 'Belisha Beacons' [introduced the previous year] to warn us where the danger of this infection exists. There may be more potential danger from an infected fellow-passenger while riding in a crowded train or omnibus than there is from the risk of accident on the journey.

He sets the facts out in a comprehensive and impartial manner, aided by numerous tables of figures, for politicians to read and draw their own conclusions, without pushing any particular point of view. Yet his reference to the National Insurance Act of 1911 sets out the key factors already known to affect health more widely (not just in the case of TB):

(a) 'Conditions or nature of employment,
(b) bad housing or insanitary conditions,
(c) insufficient or contaminated water supply, or
(d) ... health of workers in factories, workshops, mines, quarries or other industries, ... public health or the housing of the working classes...'

Of course, these factors were all agreed by the Liberals, the government which passed the 1911 Act, including Lloyd George, David Davies, Winston Churchill who was a cabinet member and president of the Board of Trade, and William Beveridge who Churchill had headhunted as a civil servant for the Board of Trade to lead on his specialist subject of unemployment insurance.

Next, from 1911 to 1935, John himself had done the statistical work to understand the root causes for the WNMA's work tackling TB and refine the list. These were not just guesses into what might be the causes, but hard facts learned from the effect of the different approaches tried out in South Wales over the years. Similarly, Beveridge had hard facts about causes of poverty in London, from working at Toynbee Hall in the East End, where he worked with Beatrice and Sidney Webb and other social reformers in the Fabian Society.

Now compare these to the Five Giants in the Beveridge Report of 1942:[21]

(a) Want – tackled by a minimum income safety net, so that everyone can afford basics such as food and basic clothing, whatever their employment or unemployment status

(b) Disease – tackled by a national health service, free at the point of use, including public health initiatives such as ensuring safe and healthy conditions at work, ensuring a safe and sufficient water supply

(c) Ignorance – tackled by national provision of education – which is also a good opportunity to give children and young people free school meals to tackle Want, teach children and young people about health and hygiene to tackle Disease and Squalor, and give children and young people skills for future jobs to tackle Idleness and Want

(d) Squalor – tackled by national provision of good quality council housing to replace slum housing, with a good water supply, and a minimum income so that people can afford cleaning materials

(e) Idleness – tackled by national control of unemployment levels and close to full employment for those able to work

We can see that the two lists originate from the same principles and therefore the same deep experience and policy work by the Welsh TB group, based on John's statistics. Beveridge had administratively organised the different policy streams into what would become different post-war government departments: social security, health, education, housing and employment.

On the business case side, John suggests that if there were fewer working days lost to sickness, then this would be of substantial economic benefit – more working days spent healthy means more goods and services produced, which means more salaries for employees and more profit for employers. It also means more contributions to National Health Insurance, which means better support for those who are still sick or have a disability.

On the statistical side, John also suggests at several points in the article that complete national morbidity figures (statistics on everyone who has a disease and which diseases they have) would be helpful. This is because these figures were needed in order to take action on the appropriate diseases when setting up national health services, and to see the effect of such services on reducing the incidence of the diseases that it was being set up to tackle, so that different approaches could be piloted and then rolled out with certainty of their effectiveness.

At one point he mentions Jarrow as having the highest average death rate from TB over a 12-year period – this could be seen as a subtle political prod, helping readers to make the connection between TB and unemployment. After years of high unemployment in the area, the main employer in

Jarrow, Palmer's Shipyard, had closed a year before, meaning there were now hardly any jobs. The political pressure was building and the following year, 1936, would see the Jarrow Crusade protest against unemployment and poverty in the town, led by local Labour MP Ellen Wilkinson on a long hunger march to London. The march hugely increased public awareness that people were being affected by unemployment and poverty not of their own making, and helped soften attitudes to support people as recommended by the Beveridge Report.

John's mention of Bermondsey as having one of the highest death rates from TB in London would have been well known. Ada Salter, the first female mayor of a London borough, and her husband Dr Alfred Salter MP were already very active in the community. Alfred Salter himself already had TB from working as a doctor in the slums. They had set up local health services to tackle the high TB rate and were already building one of the first free TB sanatoriums in London, which opened in 1937. In the same building, 74 years later, I took my daughter to a baby group where she met her best friend. When the full NHS started in 1948, Bermondsey was one of the places, like Tredegar in South Wales, which already had extensive health provision.

In the discussion printed at the end of John's paper, a comment from an audience member that King Edward had said if tuberculosis were preventable, why not prevent it, was a very helpful reminder to the right-wingers in the audience that there was royal support for this. And that was the original reason the Welsh National Memorial Association was set up too, to honour King Edward VII.

In 1939 John explained what happened as a result of his paper:

> The disclosures in that paper as to the position of the Welsh Counties in relation to tuberculosis stirred the friendly societies of the country into active movement. The National Conference at Folkestone in the same year referred the subject to their Executive Committee; the Executive interviewed the Minister of Health regarding it and suggested that it would be of advantage for representatives of the Conference to confer with his advisers as to what action could usefully be taken to improve the conditions disclosed. I was the spokesman of that deputation and Sir Kingsley Wood [Minister of Health] said he was much indebted for the statement on a matter of great national importance. He agreed that the figures submitted were very disturbing and promised to ask his Chief Medical Officer to let him have a report on those figures.[22]

Returning to John's landmark year of 1935, in September he attended the National Conference of Friendly Societies at Folkestone. Speakers included Sir Kingsley Wood, minister of health, and Sir Walter Kinnear. John was elected upon the executive committee of the Conference at the head of the poll. He had also been at the head of the poll for the Directors of the Oddfellows that year. Both implied he would become the leader soon, but he couldn't do both jobs at once. Which way would he choose to go?[23]

Grandparenthood

The same year, 1935, also marked another milestone in John's life, at the age of 61: his first grandchild, David, was born. The family were living on the same street as John's office, Arthur Street.

In 1933, John and Edith's middle daughter Doris had married Dr James Stewart, immortalised to us all as 'Uncle Jim'. Another Irish doctor in the family, Uncle Jim was no doubt a great source of information and debate as John sought to promote national healthcare provision. He was still fondly remembered in our family every time we went to the beach at Ynyslas in mid Wales, where my grandparents met. 'Uncle Jim always said swimming in the sea is very healthy. If you have a cut you should swim in the sea as the salt water sterilizes it,' my dad would inform us.

Jim Stewart was the GP in Montgomery from 1926 until the mid-1960s. He started as a sole practitioner. As the practice expanded, he took on Dr Humphreys as a partner in 1948. Other doctors later joined them too. From the 1930s to 1960s, Jim was also the medical officer for the Forden Institution, a mental hospital run by the local authority, at the site of the former Forden Workhouse. This later became Brynhyfryd Mental Hospital after the NHS was set up in 1948.

I can imagine John working away determinedly in his efforts to build a national health service, and meeting often with his son-in-law Jim, as the local GP. The two of them were likely to be in very serious discussion about death rates and what could be done about them, with the mood occasionally lightened by his daughter Doris proudly popping in to show off the new baby in his pram. The three adults would have laughed and joked about whether little David would grow up to become a doctor like his daddy.

David was soon followed by two more grandchildren, Maureen, born in 1937, and Peter, in 1944. John's son Edward – my grandfather – was 24 years old in 1935 and was training at his father's firm of solicitors. He was very good looking and always sought after by the girls. Edward's older sisters were hoping to matchmake him with one of their friends. John's reference comparing traffic accidents to deaths by TB in his journal article may well have been inspired by his son at this time, as Edward loved to drive fast and lost his front teeth in a car crash in the 1930s.

Sidney Pryce, John's partner, was by then 73 years old and had passed on his share in the firm to his son, Vaughan Pryce. Vaughan followed in Sidney's footsteps as town clerk for Montgomery. My dad and his brothers remembered often being taken to see Uncle Vaughan in his office. He was always surrounded by piles of paper and had to scrabble around to find sweets which he had set aside as treats for them. In those days sugar was rationed, so Vaughan would have been taking this out of his own ration.

The eldest of my dad's brothers, Angus Snow, was born in 1936, so he would have started visiting the office then, with his mother, Sydney. I'm sure Sydney did not miss any chance to let Sidney and John Tomley know about her husband's career success, after her father Sidney had disapproved of him: Jack Snow was now captain of the *Queen Mary* and sharing his captain's table with famous names such as Einstein.

John and Sidney were extremely proud of their two grandsons the same age, David and Angus, so encouraged them to play together, and they went to primary school together. This is how the Snow boys got to know Uncle Jim. When the boys' mother, Sydney, died of cancer in 1944, and their father Jack had to go back to sea until 1947 in order to complete post-war movements of troops and refugees around the world, Uncle Jim helped out by taking the Snow boys on holiday to the seaside at Ynyslas. There, they would play on the beach with David and his siblings and their Tomley cousins. Eventually the youngest Snow brother, my dad, was introduced to David's younger Tomley cousin, my mum.

Sydney was one of the last young adults in Montgomery to die before the introduction of the NHS in 1948. With the cost of her medical care, and the long-term cost of childcare for four small boys, the family soon went from well to do to cash strapped. Uncle Vaughan helped where he could, yet was affected by the stress of his younger sister's death and died himself eight years later. Soon, people in similar situations would be supported with free medical care from the NHS.

Call Back Yesterday

While I was researching John Tomley's life at the National Library of Wales, I looked at some tea towels in the National Library's gift shop as I was heading upstairs. There was a tea towel of a map of Wales, made up of the names of famous authors. I looked at Montgomery, and there was the name of Geraint Goodwin. I knew that name as a distant relative. Sidney Pryce's wife Mary's cousin was a Goodwin. I also remembered a book on our bookshelves at home, as a child, with the name Geraint Goodwin. On looking him up, I was astounded to see he had died young, of TB, and was a WNMA patient. The National Library of Wales had reprinted his most acclaimed book, *The Heyday in the Blood*, about a village in mid Wales, hence the tea towel.

Geraint Goodwin originally came from the village of Llanllwchaearn, near Newtown. After school, he moved to London and became a journalist. In 1930, at the age of 27, he was diagnosed with TB and spent several months in a sanatorium in London. In 1935, at 32, he wrote a novel about his experience, *Call Back Yesterday*, dedicated to his baby daughter Myfanwy – who was a schoolfriend of my dad.

Goodwin's book was helpful in popularizing the issues surrounding TB and creating public awareness. *Call Back Yesterday* is no longer in print, and I would have had to go the National Library of Wales to find it, so it was fortunate that I was already there that day.

The book tells the story of how a boy moves from a low-income home in Wales to London, assisted by his uncle, an MP in London, who secures him a job as a journalist. He then ends up in hospital in London, and gives us an intimate picture of the TB ward:

> I had lain there for days, not seeing anyone, eyes fixed on the ceiling, lying there like an animal behind the bars. I could only glare – at the doctors, the sisters, the nurses, the medical students. They were always asking questions... Sometimes I could feel my spirit rising from somewhere deep within me – smouldering somewhere within the dead ashes of my being and blowing into a thin flame. It was then that I would want to rush out as I was – where, it did not matter – to rush out somewhere and be free...
>
> Old Jarvie had been there longer than anyone remembered. He was going to die, of course, and since everyone knew it, he assumed some sort of importance among us... It was the first man who was going to die I had ever seen. I would watch him reading his daily newspaper every morning and marvel. All that information – where was it going to? What was the use of it?

107

> But Old Jarvie knew himself... He feared that they would
> move him, if he did not die in the meantime, to the infirmary
> (which, as everyone knows, is a workhouse), and this was his
> great regret...[24]

Gareth, the fictional Geraint, leaves the hospital and is taken from the London hospital to a sanatorium by the sea on the south coast:

> Here were the gates of this bare and desolate place... It was like
> one of those vast municipal cemeteries, a lifeless wilderness,
> with its trim walks and gravel paths and foolish flowers...
> 'Keep off the grass' was pegged out every few yards...
>   I lay there listening to the sea. What a small world I lived in
> after all. That outside world now seemed far off and remote,
> and I did not know when I should get back to it.

At the end of the book, on the last page, the fictional hero, Gareth, feels that he is cured from TB. In real life, Geraint was not so lucky. Despite treatment from the WNMA at one of their sanatoriums in Wales, he died before he reached the age of 40.

The description of a young adult facing early death is rare to find these days, yet Geraint's story was tragically common in the 1930s. While many things have been superseded by the NHS, there is a key issue which still applies to people facing early death today: a complete lack of NHS-funded counselling or any kind of talking opportunities for people facing early death.

The appetite for insurance

By the end of 1935, John had already taken his call for a TB inquiry to MPs through Clement Davies, and to the medical profession through his journal article. Voters need to agree too though. John spoke about TB in Wales at the WNMA's annual general meeting and decided it was time to rally the millions of members of the Oddfellows, through an article in the *Oddfellows Magazine* reporting his speech. Other Oddfellows leaders soon took up John's call to action too. The same edition also reported Director Ballard speaking on the issue at the Oddfellows' South Wales and Monmouthshire conference.[25]

On its front page – headlined 'The appetite for insurance' – it noted a change in public thinking which might help to lead to solutions for TB and other issues. People were moving towards the idea of full state National Insurance and National Health Insurance for everybody:

> Twenty-five years ago every snob in the land was anxious to keep out of National Insurance. To-day every sensible person is anxious to be in... To be under the State umbrella even though its protection against the storms is exceedingly limited, is now a general desire.

In February 1936, meanwhile, John handed updated figures about TB mortality directly to the minister of health, now covering 1934. This time it was taken a little more seriously. Memos between Dr MacNalty and Dr T.W. Wade, one of the government medical officers based at the Welsh Board of Health, are noted in the Ministry of Health files. MacNalty wrote to Wade:

> Mr Tomley recently handed to the Minister a table of figures relating to tuberculosis mortality in certain areas of England and Wales during the five years 1930-34... May I have your observations upon the Welsh figures, and the suggested reasons for this high tuberculosis mortality ... I am aware that an inquiry into this subject is to be made by the General Purposes Committee of the Welsh National Memorial Association, but both you and Dr Powell may already have views upon the subject which will be helpful to me in preparing my report to the Minister on these figures.

The reply came back from Dr Wade the following month:

> Our figures would improve if the standard of living of the people could be raised and the women were better instructed in domestic science, the relative values of food stuffs and the methods of preparation of food...

The accompanying papers went on to explain the high TB rates in Wales. Some parts were rather obstructive, for example criticising John for using crude death rates rather than standardised death rates where the age distribution of people in each area had been adjusted for. This would have been almost impossible for John to achieve himself without a team of statisticians. The way that John had arranged his figures, showing the change in death rates for each area, generally overcame this issue because each area was likely to have a similar age distribution of people from year to year – industrial areas had more working age adults, rural areas had more children and older people.

Also, it was apparently 'usual to consider mainly the respiratory form of the disease' when looking at statistics – John had looked at all forms of TB. Looked at from today's point of view, of course all forms of the disease should be looked at together as they are likely to be linked.

TB rates being higher in the west of Wales compared to the east is blamed on race. Due to the mountains separating people, 'there has been little intermixture of races, the mountains acting as a barrier to easy intercourse and it has been held by some that the Celt is specially vulnerable to tuberculosis.' This is directly comparable to the way that people think minorities excluded from health services today are simply more likely to suffer health issues due to their race, gender, disability or neurodiversity. Of course, with the benefit of hindsight we know it is because there were no doctors there, as well as no sanitation. Silicosis from slate mine work was also blamed, even though many of the deaths were in young women who would not have been miners.

Elsewhere, explanations are given which are circular. Apparently the TB mortality in Glamorgan was high because 'the death rate for that county shows practically no tendency to fall', i.e., deaths are high because deaths are high.

Facing up to the Giants

Yet other parts of the papers held the keys which would later unlock the mystery of TB death rates. The shadows of the Five Giants were starting to be seen at the Ministry of Health level. These papers were later used for the Welsh TB inquiry. Passages in the files were underlined in pencil, probably by the TB inquiry reviewers:

> Life is hard and frugal... it is probable that the main predisposing factors have been poor diet and the backward sanitary conditions. It is believed that there is more ill-health among the people of West Wales than among the people in most parts of the country. A study of the statistics of mortality from all causes gives strong support to this view...
>
> [In Glamorgan] there seems little doubt that the distressed economic conditions are in large measure responsible for this unfavourable position...

> Reduced incomes through the depression in the coal industry have caused many families to live under conditions bordering on starvation. In such circumstances it is not surprising that little or no progress is being made in reducing the pulmonary tuberculosis death-rate for the county...

John had cleverly organised a pincer movement so that Dr Powell, principal medical officer of the WNMA, would respond strongly in favour of a TB inquiry. Dr Powell responded to the Ministry of Health doctors a few days later in March 1936, demolishing the race theory. From his vantage point in Wales itself and with direct connections to the grassroots medical services, he could see things the Ministry of Health staff in London could not see, despite their medical training. Dr Powell could see the outlines of the Five Giants clearly.

> At its meeting only last week the Medical Committee suggested that the mass of material now available, largely owing to Mr Tomley's efforts, deserved to critically analysed and worked up by experts in order that its real statistical significance should be ascertained, and I was instructed in fact to put this suggestion before the Department for its consideration... a letter from Professor Picken (of which I enclose a copy) was circulated in which he points out that the incidence and mortality of tuberculosis is only a part of the general health and medical problem of Wales. [Picken said:]
> 'The main factor, however, in my opinion, lies in the interplay of forces of infection and resistance, infection being exceedingly high and concentrated in the small, insalubrious houses of north and west Wales, where family infection is transmitted with great facility and where nearly all the households in some of the counties are closely related and in constant and intimate contact with each other. Resistance, on the other hand, tends to be very low in country places... The lesson of Mr Tomley's investigation is, to my mind, that the campaign against tuberculosis should be directed, as far as possible, against the infected home as a unit.'

Powell agreed, and wrote that there were (underlining again from the later inquiry) 'excessive opportunities for infection rather than... a lack of resisting power, whether due to heredity or to an adverse environment'.

He added that other factors included young women having to enter 'the hurly-burly of industrial competition' – i.e., work in factories after the loss of so many men in the First World War – and 'overshadowing all, the industrial depression with its repercussions on physique, nutrition, and morale'. But there were solutions requiring joined-up thinking:

> As to how these rates could be reduced, the efforts of the Association should be aimed primarily at controlling infection by (1) the provision of an increasing number of beds, until waiting-lists are a thing of the past, and (2) a much more generous provision for the follow-up of cases, the search for contacts, and the stringent domiciliary supervision of the families of tuberculous patients... The support of general practitioners should also be enlisted in the search for suspects and in the methods of home prevention, and closer co-operation secured with the Maternity and Child Welfare and School Medical Services.

In Picken's letter attached, his final paragraph was highlighted in its entirety by the later TB inquiry reviewers:

> There is, then, a general health and medical problem of Wales, of which the incidence and mortality of tuberculosis are only a part. We shall lose perspective if we forget that tuberculosis mortality is rather a measure of public health progress than a separate problem by itself.

This proved to be a key driving factor in the TB inquiry, which was widened from the medical treatment of TB to the wider prevention of TB and many other diseases. The Five Giants were now firmly in the doctors', statisticians' and politicians' sights.

The only way the factors of 'poverty, overcrowding and undernutrition' (in the words of the same Dr Chapman who had dismissed John's statistics the year before) could be removed was by removing all factors together – exactly the point of tackling the Five Giants together which would later be highlighted in the Beveridge Report.

By April 1936, Clem Davies was on the case again. A Ministry of Health memo notes:

> Mr Clement Davies K.C., M.P., came to see the Minister yesterday and asked, among other things, what is the

present position in regard to the enquiries which the Minister undertook to have made in reply to the representations made by Mr J. Tomley at the deputation from the National Conference of Friendly Societies...

This was answered in pen below by Dr MacNalty: 'Mr Wilkinson – I have had reports prepared on this subject by Dr Wade, Senior Medical Officer Welsh Board of Health, Dr D. A. Powell, Principal Medical Officer Welsh National Insurance Assocn, and by Dr Chapman, SMO for Tuberculosis of this dept...' Dr MacNalty asked his colleague Dr Chapman to review the report he was compiling. Chapman was starting to come round from his previous opposition and was particularly convinced by the evidence from Dr Picken:

Dr Picken's letter to Dr Powell seems to me to touch the heart of the matter. I have long felt that if in a number of areas the mortality from respiratory tuberculosis could be considered not alone but in relation to mortality from certain other diseases especially respiratory diseases a degree of parallelism would probably be found. This would indicate the operation of a common factor and would lead to the study of mortality of which tuberculosis was only one item.

The reason for Dr Chapman's earlier resistance becomes clear: workload. It 'would require more time and clerical assistance than is available', although he did have 'a partial and preliminary investigation in hand'.

Things seemed to be looking promising from this paperwork. Yet I was astounded to discover that the final Ministry of Health internal report, completed towards the end of April 1936, was another stitch-up. What on earth had happened?

John Tomley's statistical methods were openly criticized again. MacNalty wrote:

These observations have raised some doubt as to the real statistical significance of Mr Tomley's figures. The figures are considered too small to lend themselves for statistical analysis. The Medical Committee of the Welsh National Memorial Association has suggested that the mass of material now available, largely owing to Mr Tomley's efforts, deserved to be critically analysed and worked up by experts in order that its real statistical significance should be ascertained.

MacNalty said that 'the general influence of contact infection, of certain occupations and of poverty, overcrowding and insanitary conditions in causing a high rate of tuberculosis was demonstrated many years ago, but it is often difficult or impossible to ascertain why mortality should differ in two specific areas', dismissing John's data and again raising the idea of 'less resistance and less immunity to tuberculosis in the inhabitants of these areas', linked to the discredited ideas of race and gender. And then he really wields the knife:

> It will thus be seen that Mr Tomley as an amateur of vital statistics is dealing with a problem from a superficial standpoint which has engaged the study and unremitting attention of Government departments and workers in tuberculosis for over half a century. In fact, his crude figures hardly merit serious attention by expert statisticians and he has already received more notice and courtesy than they deserve.

He concluded:

> We are well aware of the wide variations in the mortality from tuberculosis in the different areas of England and Wales; the subject has been extensively studied by officers of my Department for a number of years... I understand also that an inquiry into the subject of high tuberculosis mortality in Wales is to be made by the General Purposes Committee of the Welsh National Memorial Association which already have Mr Tomley's figures before them.
>
> You and Mr Tomley may rest assured that we are continually cooperating with Local Authorities and the Welsh National Memorial Association in further measures for the prevention and treatment of tuberculosis, and that, while the high mortality from the disease in certain areas is still a matter of concern, the general and progressive decline in the incidence and mortality from tuberculosis in England and Wales is of encouraging import.

In other words, don't worry your little heads about these very complicated statistics which are a matter for real health leaders like us. The letter was duly written and signed in May 1936 by Kingsley Wood, minister of health, and sent to Clem to pass on to John.

So how had this stitch-up come about?

The first issue of course was the workload issue discussed earlier in the Ministry of Health files. A stitch-up like this meant that no further work had to be done, saving everyone's limited time.

It sounds like it wasn't just the workload issue either. The tone of the report is very clear that John's statistics were 'Not invented here'. This is a key issue that still dogs NHS senior management today when patient views are being put across – as patients are not yet welcome to be senior managers in the NHS and become part of the 'Here' group, everything patients say automatically falls into the 'Not invented here' category. It then has a tendency to be overlooked.

Another issue would have been the political ramifications of giving the public data which could lead to people calling for an end to poverty. The government of the day had no money to resolve any of these issues. Unemployment and inflation was high and taxes could not be increased to overcome this. It was hoped that the economy would recover and there would be a trickle-down effect to solve poverty. In a few years' time, things would be all right and people would be employed... Yet, as the economist Keynes was pointing out at the time, 'In the long run we are all dead.' There was more to government than just letting workers be crushed by each roll of the economic cycle, from boom to bust and back again. Yet the government of the day was scared to admit it in case they lost an election.

The Five Giants had been within tackling distance, yet were now vanishing into the mist once again.

'Sit on this'

John was not deterred, however. The very next month, June 1936, he wrote to Clem Davies again, asking for the TB statistics for 1935. Seeing as the Ministry of Health claimed to have its finger on the pulse with its own TB statistics, surely they should be prepared to share them with other health leaders such as the WNMA board? Clem wrote to the Ministry of Health to ask.

Dr MacNalty at the ministry was offended when asked to advise what reply should be made. A handwritten note under the memo reads: 'Is not the reply that the figures are not yet available? We cannot give Mr Tomley priority over our own Annual Reports.' Dr Chapman wrote underneath: 'I understand from Dr Stocks... that a preliminary study of the S. Wales figures shows evidence of some deterioration but sit on this till the complete figures are ready.'

So a further cover-up of the worsening situation for young people with TB in South Wales meant that no one actually running health services on the ground could take prompt action to tackle the extra deaths. John was a pioneer of big data and this shows exactly why that is needed today – datasets that are publicly available, for free, on a timely basis, and in spreadsheet form so that anyone can analyse them in order to improve life for us all.

In July 1936, there was suspicion over the cover-up and questions were being asked in the House of Commons. The Ministry of Health files show that Jim Griffiths MP (Labour, Llanelli) asked the Minister of Health

> if there has been any improvement in the mortality rate from tuberculosis in the industrial areas of South Wales, particularly in the age groups of 15-25 years and 25-30 years to which attention was called in the Report of the Chief Medical Officer of the Ministry of Health for the year 1933; and whether he will direct the attention of the Unemployment Assistance Board to the Report of the Chief Medical Officer and ask the Board to bear it in mind when fixing scales and conditions of assistance to unemployed persons in those areas.

Sir Kingsley Wood replied that the death rates from TB in Wales showed 'some improvement during that period, though emigration from this area may render interpretation of the figures... somewhat difficult'. Griffiths queried the 'improvement' but Wood stood his ground.

By August 1936, Clem was again pressing the Ministry of Health for the TB statistics John had requested. Eventually the grudging reply came back in the files that John could have the preliminary statistics as it was likely to be some time before they would be published by the registrar general.

The WNMA battles on

In the meantime, the WNMA fight continued to raise awareness of TB and its causes, based on John's statistics. In May 1936, the WNMA's new medical committee chair Dr John Jones said 'that he had a scheme whereby tuberculosis in Wales in 10 years' time would be as rare as typhoid fever today'. He added that 'we are not doing what we should for our health services' and that the only way to cure tuberculosis was to spend money. The statistics, again supported by Professor Picken, showed there was 'a general health and medical problem of Wales on which the evidence and mortality of tuberculosis are only a part'. As usual, John was on hand with the data – here pointing out that male TB mortality was 30 per cent higher than among women.

The *Western Mail* also reported that 'A clash between the Welsh Board of Health and the King Edward VII Memorial Association appeared imminent' over 'proposed expenditure of £3,500 on renewing the engineering plant at the South Wales Sanatorium'. The supervising engineer had warned that 'in the event of a breakdown the institution would be paralysed', especially over winter.[26]

June 1936 brought some seemingly negative news for John at the Oddfellows' Annual Moveable Conference in Douglas. After being tipped for the top, to be grand master of the Oddfellows, he withdrew his application in favour of another candidate, Mr Toogood.[27] What did this mean? Has he given up on his fight against T.B.?

It may be that John already had his eye on the bigger prize of leading the whole friendly society movement in order to use his TB statistics to call for a national inquiry. That call had already been discussed at the WNMA meeting John was at earlier. Perhaps Mr Toogood had offered to help him as long as John backed him for grand master of the Oddfellows? The tradition was always that whoever was elected deputy leader then was elected leader the following year.

In the same month, John was at the committee looking at prescription costs for Wales, which he chaired. There was a statistical table of average cost per prescription and average cost per person, which seemed to be new information the committee hadn't had before. I suspect this was John's doing.

There is a pattern to all these new statistics being produced that were never before available. Why was John the first to produce so many statistical analyses? Was he the only person in the history of health that ever thought about doing it? The answer probably lies in new technology of the time. The newfangled adding and calculating machines, the mechanical precursor of the modern calculator, were widely sold from about 1909 onwards in America. They then caught on in Britain too. Eventually they became cheap enough for a local health commissioner to buy, which is probably when John invested in one for his office. He always loved to be an early adopter of new technology, and we know he had already bought one of the first cameras in his town as well as one of the first dictation machines which burned a wax record, which I inherited from him. The new calculating machine would have meant John could add a list of statistical figures for different areas. He could also divide figures on the machine to get percentages, instead of the old fashioned and very time-consuming method of long division.

In July 1936, the annual meeting of the WNMA took place. John presented his report with new figures for TB deaths in rural Wales, ending with a rousing call to action:

> Are we to act fearlessly and effectively as a Fire Bridge in extinguishing this conflagration, or are we content to be merely a Salvage Corps dealing with the debris and the ruins instead of fighting the living and devastating flames?[28]

The meeting also heard about progress at the Sully Hospital, which now had 1,816 beds for TB patients, and plans for a 'proposed new hospital at Singleton Park, Swansea, with accommodation of 250 beds and costing about £200,000, with annual running costs of about £37,000'. A newspaper report added:

> In other words, infection in the country villages is chiefly met with in the home and tends to be intense; whereas in the non-infected families working in the open and living in tubercle-free, though overcrowded, houses no resistance is acquired, and inter-marriage or other intimate contact with infected neighbours may later on produce devastating results.
>
> Professor Cummins says that the lesson to be derived from the investigations of Mr J.E. Tomley is that the campaign against tuberculosis, should be directed, as far as possible, against the infected home as a unit.[29]

In August, John spoke about his TB statistics at an event discussing public health services in Wales at the Welsh School of Social Service at Llandrindod Wells. The main speaker, Professor Ralph Picken, presented an academic paper making the argument for a centrally managed national health service. The Welsh councils were too small, and found it hard to provide an efficient service. He recommended that all hospitals should be organised into a full state-managed national health service, explaining that the Welsh Consultative Council on Medical and Allied Services had reviewed health provision in 1920–21 and had suggested a national health service comprising hospitals, laboratories and regional health services:

> No doubt its members were impressed with the outstanding success of the Welsh National Memorial Association in the

treatment of cases of tuberculosis from all parts of Wales. Here they had an organization which showed that Wales was workable as an executive unit which had built up a service better, of its kind, than that in almost every other part of the United Kingdom.

Picken explained that the suggestion of a national health service had been 'too ambitious, too revolutionary' at the time in the early 1920s, and had not been able to be put into practice due to a lack of resources. Now, in the mid 1930s, it was an idea whose time had come.[30]

On the same page, the newspaper reported that David Lloyd George was now a shopkeeper and had opened a farm shop to sell his farm's produce. At Westminster, the Welsh Wizard was no more. John and David Davies were now the most senior Welsh health leaders. It was up to them to push forward on securing the Welsh TB inquiry by the Minister of Health, to prove the need for a full NHS.

Before the year was over, John was elected vice-president of the National Conference of Friendly Societies, the second highest role in the overall friendly societies movement, which was reported in a number of newspapers across the UK, including *The Western Mail*.[31]

The fight starts in earnest

John himself explained in the *Oddfellows Magazine* what happened next with his TB statistical work. As a result of his journal paper on TB and visit to the minister of health, he had persuaded the Association of Welsh Insurance Committees, where he was a member of the executive committee, to take action:

> This Association has always been greatly concerned with the subject of Tuberculosis because its constituent committees are responsible for the medical treatment of all the hundreds of thousands of insured persons throughout Wales.
>
> We asked for a conference with the Welsh National Memorial Association to discuss the remedial measures which might be found advisable. That conference was held at Shrewsbury under the Presidency of Lord Davies in December, 1936... The Conference decided in favour of a more intensive examination and follow-up of tuberculosis cases and their contacts, the improvement in many areas

of such directly preventive measures as disinfection, the systematic obtaining and recording of the basic data as regards patients and contacts, the provision, on a national basis, of 'after care' for persons suffering from tuberculosis and their families, the provision of additional beds and the nucleus of a Village Settlement in Wales [for people to recover longer term from TB].[32]

Yet when the WNMA tried to increase their services to tackle TB more effectively, a fight broke out. The local authorities did not want to fund the services that were needed, such as new buildings and more doctors and nurses.

It was a big political problem that capital expenditure on new buildings had to be fully charged in the year the building was built, causing the local authorities to bear a large cost in their budgets that year. This is a key political factor that has shaped the NHS. This is why accountancy rules today allow the capital cost to be spread over the many years that a building is in use, up to 50 years.

There was also a lack of systems thinking at the time. People who could see long term, like John and David Davies, knew that to eradicate TB would be a long-term fight and they needed a lot more resources at their disposal, including not only a comprehensive national health service with more hospitals, clinics, doctors and nurses, but also decent homes and safe water supplies for all areas of Wales, as well as a minimum income so that people could afford a reasonable diet, basic clothes and cleaning materials. The councillors from the local authorities at the time could not see this longer-term goal. All they could see was their taxpayers were not being cured of TB by the time they faced re-election.

In systems thinking, delay is a key concept that we must understand and build into systems diagrams so that we can explain to people why there is sometimes a timing difference between taking action and seeing the result. If the councillors who fought progress (as we'll see in the article below) could have known that TB would be pretty much eradicated in the UK when the BCG vaccine was introduced sixteen years later, they might have been more supportive. Yet sixteen years is a short time in people's lifetimes and a long time in politics – councillors might still have been more worried about being re-elected than about curing TB. This is one of the reasons why the NHS was purposefully set up outside local authority control.

In January 1937, the *Western Mail & South Wales News* ran a story under this headline:

SPEEDING-UP FIGHT AGAINST TUBERCULOSIS IN WALES
Plans Include New Hospital and Village Settlement

Authorities Oppose £500,000 Estimate for Next Five Years

The report covered a conference in Cardiff between the WNMA and relevant authorities to resolve issues before a formal consultation with the minister of health. David (now Lord) Davies presided and the issues under discussion were listed as:

1. The provision on a national basis of 'after-care' for persons suffering for tuberculosis and their families.
2. The continuation of the association's policy of accepting financial responsibility for tuberculous cases in public assistance institutions.
3. The provision of additional beds, including a hospital at Swansea, and the nucleus of a village settlement in Wales.
4. The more intensive examination and follow-up of tuberculosis cases and their contacts; the improvement in many areas of such directly preventive measures as disinfection; the systematic obtaining and recording of basic data as regards patients and contacts, and generally the position and progress of the Welsh National anti-tuberculosis campaign.
5. The suggested revision of the basis upon which local authorities make their contributions.

Councillors from Flintshire attending this conference, which the lord mayor of Cardiff called 'the most important in the history of the association', described the estimated five-year cost of £500,000 as 'alarming' and issued a formal objection. Lord Davies spoke of the long-term challenges:

'We have tried many experiments,' he said, 'and spent a considerable amount of money, erected a number of hospitals, and secured the services of eminent medical men, but we must admit that, in spite of these investigations and research and of all our efforts, we have not been able to make the progress we had expected 20 years ago.

From the experience we have gained we are now in the position to undertake larger and more comprehensive measures in order to try once more to get down to the very root of things and try to eradicate this scourge. Given all the facilities which are essential in carrying on, we shall succeed.

But Flintshire persisted in their 'strong opposition', argued on the basis that TB services accounted for 50 per cent of their health service spend while the disease was 'responsible for only seven per cent of the deaths in Wales'. Alderman Waterhouse of Flintshire also 'suggested this was not the time to embark on a large building programme, and he moved that the estimate of £200,000 for a new hospital at Swansea be deleted' and was seconded by Denbighshire council. Of course, as we have heard before, TB was the biggest cause of death in young people, and was a preventable cause of death, so it was in reality proportionate.

In Flintshire, for example, the local council's health service spend was only £22,000 per year. This is £1.6m today, far less than would be spent on the NHS now, which is in the order of £100m or more per county per year – more than 100 times as much. No wonder this tiny spend in 1937 was having very little effect on TB or other health issues.

Dr John Jones, chairman of the WNMA's medical committee, responded firmly:

If you are going to measure the lives of men, women and children in the terms of pounds, shillings, and pence you are never going to do away with this scourge. You are bound to spend the money, and we are pledged to build the hospital at Swansea.

He also warned that there was a waiting list of 335 people in Swansea. The debate continued, and some councillors at least seemed to understand the case for long-term thinking. Alderman John Donovan of Cardiff argued 'if they were to look at the £ s d first and not give the necessary thought to the disease they were not going to get very far', and his colleague G. Fred Evans reminded everyone that since the WNMA started, TB deaths in Wales had been reduced by a third.

Lord Davies wrapped things up, saying the campaign was an investment, and 'We must eradicate this disease so that we will not have to go to authorities year after year for their contributions', and finished by pleading that 'when they went before the Minister of Health they should go as a united body'. It was agreed that the cost estimates should be reviewed further.[33]

The mention of a waiting list is interesting as a justification for the spend – waiting lists are still used today as a political reason to justify the need for NHS expenditure. Yet waiting lists are very bad for patients, whose condition may worsen while on them, potentially causing their death. If the system was tweaked to get rid of waiting lists, this would clearly be much better for patients.

The statistics quoted by some of the opposing councillors seem a bit suspect – they are different from the ones John had highlighted in his paper for the Royal Sanitary Institute and underplay the true level of TB, as well as ignoring that TB mainly affected younger people, so was more urgent to tackle than causes of death due to old age.

Taking it to the government

In February 1937, the Ministry of Health correspondence files show that John wrote to Clem Davies with more statistics following the WNMA meeting, thanking him for his latest letter and saying 'I… am glad that you will be able to read the Report I sent you of the Conference at Cardiff on the 29th ultimo as it will give you a good idea of the difficulty in persuading these good people [the local authorities] to help themselves.'

The following week, John wrote again to Clem:

> Tuberculosis Mortality – The enclosed notes will, I think, supply the 'brief' which you asked me to submit to you on this subject when we last met in London. My manuscript has been in Cardiff for some time and the Memorial Association have duplicated copies of it. If there is any amplification you would like to have from me I will endeavour to provide it, but I think the enclosed covers the ground.[34]

John later reflected on what had happened at the WNMA meeting and how Clem used it as ammunition to fight for a government investigation:

> A revised [cost] estimate [for WMNA activities] was prepared at the request of a conference of the contributing authorities was submitted to a second conference of those authorities at Shrewsbury in March, 1937. At this latter conference, to quote from the Annual Report of the Memorial Association, 'The tone which prevailed was very different from that of

the previous conference. It appeared as though a concerted attempt, instigated and inspired from some unknown quarter, had been made in the meantime in order to discredit the Association and to repudiate its general policy by a wholesale rejection of the new proposals in the estimate.'

The... Minister of Health confined his consideration to the non-controversial part of the Association's estimates, representing substantially the continuation of existing services. The Memorial Association would not, however, accept this solution. They stood to their guns, reaffirmed the estimates which had been presented, and asked the Minister to make a special investigation into their work, and particularly in regard to the proposals put forward in the estimates. The sequel was, in the words of Mr Clement Davies and Dr Coutts, 'The Minister appointed us as a committee for that purpose.'[35]

John had finally got his wish from the minister of health. The government's Welsh TB Inquiry was about to begin, and his local MP Clem was leading on it.

Chapter 6

'No Mean Responsibility'
1937–1939

In 1937, John finally reached the very top role in the national friendly societies movement, becoming president for the year. Now he was representing healthcare providers for 12 million working people and their families, the majority of the country. The friendly societies included the largest healthcare providers at the time, which would later be transferred to the NHS. This was because friendly societies operated nationally, whereas family doctors and hospitals tended to operate individually, so were much smaller. Also, there were a lot fewer hospital services, as most working people had no access to hospital care. Overall, this meant that John was the most influential healthcare provider leader at the time. It also happened to be the National Conference's fiftieth anniversary year in 1938, a fantastic time for a president to make a splash at the conference and push for change.

John's election was reported extensively in the national press, along with occasional photos.

The first to report was *The Scotsman*, which covered all the proceedings at the 1937 National Conference. We can see John must have rubbed shoulders with the top politicians of the day. A speech by the former Labour Party leader and pacifist George Lansbury was discussed first, followed by John's election.[1]

Lansbury took the limelight in the newspapers, with a controversial speech supporting keeping the peace with Hitler, at a time when appeasement was going out of fashion. He had met with Hitler and Mussolini and they were, apparently, very nice chaps. Let us not judge him too harshly for his speech, remembering that it was still two years before the start of the Second World War at this point. It does remind us that with all the pre-war political news, it was a wonder that John managed to get anything done with taking forward the push for better healthcare. Lansbury's departure from the Labour Party in 1935 due to his pacifism enabled the election of Clement Attlee, intended as a brief 'caretaker' leader, who ended up as Winston Churchill's deputy in the Second World War coalition government and then won the post-war election, enabling him to appoint Nye Bevan as Minister of Health and get the NHS pushed through. So the outcome wasn't all bad.

The *Western Mail & South Wales News* also reported on John's new status:

FRIENDLY SOCIETIES' PRESIDENT
Election of Mr J. E. Tomley

Mr J.E. Tomley, Montgomery, who has been elected president of the National Conference of Friendly Societies, which represents a total of 7,000,000 independents and 5,000,000 State members, was elected vice-president last year.

He has been a member of the conference for 25 years, and is the first representative for Wales to reach the presidential chair.

He is senior trustee of the Manchester Unity of Oddfellows, has been a director of the order, and was for 25 years chairman of its investigation committee.

A solicitor, Mr Tomley holds numerous legal appointments in Montgomeryshire, and has been president of the Welsh Association of National Health Insurance Committees. He was given the C.B.E. in recognition of his work on War pension bodies.[2]

Only weeks after his election, the policy and influence work John had been doing as the new president had started to bear fruit. In October, for example, the *Western Mail & South Wales News* featured a long article on TB, looking at the 'relationship between the incidence of tuberculosis in Wales and migration of the nation's healthiest youth... to English industrial centres'. John was asked for his comments and quoted extensively – while clearly being keen to let readers draw their own conclusions from the facts. ('Mr Tomley... states the problem clearly in the following interview, but does not pretend to have found a solution.') Here is John:

'That migration must be the healthy people going away for employment,' Mr Tomley said. 'Well, it leaves a larger proportion of the sickly, naturally. That's one feature, and it is terribly distressing because it concerns not merely the South Wales industrial areas but every county, with the exception of Flint. The decrease is simply awful. From Montgomery, which has a population of under 50,000, 3,000 people have been lost in seven years... This is a very big political question.

'We have a terrible experience in some of our Welsh areas on the tuberculosis problem. The Western Mail reported something I said a few weeks ago pointing out that the Welsh counties had, without exception, a far higher tuberculosis rate than the English counties...

'These figures definitely show it is time something was done in Wales to stop it. The fact that we have this vast Welsh national organization at work in our country, while England has never had anything of the kind, ought to argue we ought to have a better rate than England. Instead, we have one immensely worse.'

John presented recent data and again pointed at problems in Welsh university towns, clearly emotional about the whole subject: 'I have got thousands and thousands of figures on the problem. It is such an immense thing that it leaves me at times absolutely depressed. We are getting no further.'[3]

The following week, John was in the *Western Mail & South Wales* news again. The inquiry he had been pressing for into TB in Wales had finally been started by the minister of health and he was giving evidence. This inquiry – full name the Committee of Inquiry into the Anti-Tuberculosis Service in Wales and Monmouthshire, and which revealed the benefits of a universal national health service – was a key piece of the evidence needed for the government to set up the NHS.[4]

In a later *Oddfellows Magazine*, John talked about his work that year and his triple role in the Inquiry:

The Inquiry having been established, it devolved upon the Executive of the National Conference of Friendly Societies to prepare evidence to submit to the Commission on behalf of its vast national membership... In my capacity as President of the National Conference, that duty fell to me, but in the meantime the Association of Welsh Insurance Committees also required evidence to be submitted on behalf of their seventeen constituent committees. That task fell on my shoulders, too, and frankly, this double duty was no mean responsibility.

Representing these two organizations and also acting as a Governor of the Welsh National Memorial Association, I had to attend nearly thirty separate Sessions of the Inquiry at Cardiff and Shrewsbury and to take an active part in their deliberations throughout.[5]

Hotline to the minister

While the TB inquiry was going on, John continued to write to the minister of health. In December 1937 John wrote directly to Sir Kingsley Wood, marking the correspondence as personal to ensure it got through.

> Dear Sir Kingsley,
> I am delighted to learn that you are addressing a Public Meeting at Bangor in Caernarvonshire on January 19th next because it is the sad fact that that County proves to have the highest rate of mortality from Tuberculosis amongst all the Counties of England, Wales and Scotland during the past seven years. This will be emphasised in the evidence which I shall have to give shortly before the Committee of Inquiry into the Anti-Tuberculosis arrangements in Wales which you have very wisely set up but it occurs to me that you may find it of some advantage to have an advance copy of the statistics in question. Their preparation has been quite a big job…
>
> Some other features in which I know you are keenly interested emerge from my tables e.g. the relative position of the sea-ports, especially on the North East Coast, with regard to Tuberculosis and the wonderful improvement shown during the last few years in this respect by the Metropolitan Boroughs. When I tell you that, amongst all the 62 Counties of England and Wales, seven Welsh Counties are bunched at the top of the list in respect of Tuberculosis mortality, you will understand what a useful text for your address at Bangor my figures may supply…
>
> With all good wishes,
> Yours sincerely,
> J.E. Tomley

John's upbeat letter was not matched by the attitude shown by senior Ministry of Health staff in the accompanying memos in the files. John Rowland, John's arch-nemesis from the Welsh Board of Health, even wrote:

Mr Tomley is well known to us here as a prolific correspondent. He is, I understand, equally well known to your people at Whitehall. He should not be encouraged to write to the Minister. His correspondence would bring him to the point of interviews which we all dread here. Unfortunately he is deaf.[6]

This was a fine way to treat John, who as president of the National Association of Friendly Societies was running the largest forerunner of the NHS, representing 12 million people and their families. It shows how little the Ministry of Health had really grasped the job they needed to do at that time. It also reveals the discrimination from Oxbridge-educated civil servants against the leaders of the working people's movements at the time, including both the friendly societies and the trade union-approved societies administering national health insurance for working people.

Remember when John stood up to the Welsh Insurance Commissioners in the 1910s and 1920s and was forced to leave his job as a result, causing a national outcry by the Oddfellows? Rowland was one of the Welsh Insurance Commissioners. John and his boss at Montgomeryshire National Health Insurance Committee had also offended Rowland at a meeting in 1931, showing him up by putting forward their idea of an integrated health service. Now Rowland was taking the opportunity to get his own back.

John had the last laugh though. Thanks to the TB inquiry being kicked off by his statistics, within a decade these staff would have changed and the Ministry of Health itself would be running the new NHS. In fact, Rowland himself took early retirement shortly after the TB inquiry, possibly as a result of the controversy about his lack of action, which the report had highlighted, and this exact comment.

I thought I was the first one of John's family and friends to see this particularly rude letter. But of course, Clem Davies probably saw it too, when he looked through the Ministry of Health files as part of the TB Inquiry. And yes, when I looked again, I could see there was a pencil mark under it and a pencil question mark next to this comment in the margin, the sign of the TB inquiry reviewers.

By February 1938 John was requesting a delegation from the National Conference of Friendly Societies to the Minister of Health – just as the ministry staff had not wanted. This was, however, standard practice to communicate conference decisions each year, where they were relevant to the minister, so it could not be politely turned down.

Another memo noted:

> The Minister is receiving a deputation on the 7th March from the National Conference of Friendly Societies who are submitting a number of resolutions and also wish to refer to 'Tuberculosis in Rural Areas'. Could you let me have by Monday next a short note on this subject for inclusion in the Minister's brief.

This is followed by a handwritten reply:

> The attached general note has been prepared in consultation with Dr Chapman. Mr Tomley has been a constant correspondent in the past on the subject of tuberculosis statistics, particularly in relation to Wales, though I believe his figures are more complicated than valuable.

The note of past TB statistics for the Minister was duly prepared. In the end, John was ill on the day of the meeting, yet the rest of the group attended and his colleague Stanley Duff read a letter from John.

> Will you please... be sure to take the opportunity of thanking [Sir Kingsley] on behalf of the National Conference for setting up his Committee of Inquiry into the Anti-Tuberculosis Service in Wales? This timely action on his part is typical of the Minister's thoroughness and foresight and it will have far-reaching and beneficial results throughout the Principality... many of the causes and effects of the high Tuberculosis rates in parts of Wales are to be found in English Rural Districts too...
>   Seeing the Minister opening with a golden key the portals of what was described as 'the temple of health' in Cardiff on Tuesday last, I could not but hope and trust that he may find some similar instrument for opening the portals of health to our rural communities and it may be that the golden key or generous Treasury grants for the purpose at his hands may prove to be the solution.

So fortunately John had already seen the minister the week before at the WNMA's opening of its new headquarters. Princess Elizabeth had turned down the invitation to open the building, so David Davies thought of an even better idea. He found 'the poorest miner's wife' to represent the women, mothers and wives who had lost loved ones in the First World War – Minnie James from Dowlais, who was hailed as 'the mother of Wales'.[7]

Following the delegation to the minister, Dr MacNalty was again asked to look at some of John's points. He complains in a memo in the Ministry of Health files: 'We have dealt with his superficial statistics on several occasions... I should like to have your observations on his point about the incidence of TB in English rural districts and the need for an inquiry.'

Dr Chapman produced a report which led to the conclusion: 'In the circumstances I regard a statistical study of incidence of tuberculosis in the rural areas of individual counties as of no practical value.'[8]

The Ministry of Health files include an article about John's TB statistics written by John in the February 1939 *National Insurance Gazette* – a Ministry of Health official had been asked to prepare a statement on it before the minister's visit to South Wales at the beginning of March 1939. In the same magazine, there was an article by Mr G.W. Canter, president of the National Association of Trade Union Approved Societies, a sister organization to the National Conference of Friendly Societies where John was president. Calls for a national health service were growing from that quarter too:

> We in the past have been primarily interested in National Health Insurance. Why not, therefore, make a start by endeavouring to lay the foundation of a full and complete National Medical Service, which shall include General Practitioner Service, Specialist and Consultant and Operative Services, Hospitals and Convalescent Service, professional Nursing, Nursing Homes, etc. Surely here is a start. No one can deny the need for the co-ordination of the present conglomeration of patchwork medical services, all separately controlled, overlapping in every direction and wasteful in the extreme in administration. I have long felt that the co-ordination of these services within a National scheme would provide every medical need of the worker with little, if any, addition to the present cost.

TB inquiry: evidence sessions

By January 1938, the first day's sitting of the Committee of Inquiry into the Anti-Tuberculosis Service in Wales and Monmouthshire took place and was reported in the *Western Mail and Southern News*. This was finally the chance for the Welsh TB group led by John and David Davies to explain in public why a coordinated universal national health service was the only way to deal with TB, and therefore show that such as service should be set up, following their example of the Welsh National Memorial Association which covered the whole of Wales. David was ill on the day, and so the task fell to John.

John had transformed his statistics into maps and these took pride of place on the page, titled 'A Geographical Analysis of the Incidence of Tuberculosis Mortality in England, Wales, and Scotland during the seven years, 1930-1936'. In the days before computers this was painstaking work, both calculating the statistics and making several copies of a hand-drawn map. This was one of the first times national health statistics had been collected and mapped in this way in the newspapers, yet we can see straight away the similarity with Covid-19 maps in recent times.

The newspaper reported on David's statement to the meeting, which he was too ill to attend in person: 'he pleaded that the organisation of the association should be continued on the principle on the needs of Wales as a whole, irrespective of county or borough boundaries' and he said he regarded 'certain proposals that had been made as an attempt to break up the national character of the association's scheme':

> These proposals included the transfer of the tuberculosis officer and the dispensary service of the association to individual medical officers of health and contracting for the use of the national institutions by each local authority.

John provided his first evidence, his statistics presented in map form, and those present heard how the inquiry had come to pass, with Clement Davies and Dr Francis H. Coutts appointed to conduct it. Clem Davies reminded them that the minister of health had said 'I hope that it will do much to further this important work in Wales, because I do not think that anyone can be contented with the present position or say that no more can be done'. As well as the WNMA, numerous organizations had been invited to contribute evidence to the inquiry, including seventeen county and borough councils, the Association of Welsh Insurance Committees and various other related bodies. David Davies' statement again underlined that the essence of the WNMA 'is its national basis… that our country should be regarded as a single unit for the diagnosis and treatment of tuberculosis'. That national basis had been confirmed by

Neville Chamberlain (now prime minister) when he had been minister of health himself back in 1928. His statement also reflected on criticisms of the WNMA from some people in local authorities but only those who 'did not possess first hand knowledge and experience of the problems', and affirmed the importance of working in tandem with those local authorities. The WNMA was clear in its purpose:

> Lord Davies stated there was a wide and undefined area in relation to the prevention, treatment and eradication of tuberculosis in which the association had been expected to be the mouthpiece of the whole nation, and their anxiety was to ensure that each stage in the campaign necessary for the ultimate eradication of the scourge was energetically undertaken and pursued.

He concluded that after twenty-seven years of working together

> I believe that the same solidarity and the same determination exist in our country today, and that the vast majority of our fellow countrymen support wholeheartedly a national institution which is designed not only to rid ourselves of this terrible scourge but also to enable Wales to make her contribution as a nation to the solution of the common problem which confronts every country in the fight against this insidious and devastating disease.

Dr D.A. Powell, the WNMA's principal medical officer, reminded everyone that close contact with other TB cases was the primary cause of the disease, but we see the Five Giants looming clearly in his list of 'contributory causes': 'Malnutrition, poverty, bad housing, and overcrowding'.[9]

In a later *Oddfellows Magazine*, John talked about the proposals he helped submit to the TB inquiry:

> We stressed the desirability of early diagnosis of the disease, the thorough examination of suspected cases, their reference without delay to the tuberculosis physicians, prompt notification to medical officers of Health in compliance with the regulations, and ascertainment of the incidence of tuberculosis in the various areas as revealed by the Registers which each authority is required to keep...

> We also ask[ed] for the clearing of the long list of
> Tuberculosis patients requiring institutional treatment which
> continually exists in Wales by the provision of additional
> institutional accommodation and the setting up of a
> colony in Wales such as proves so successful in England...
> This recommendation met with strong and well-organized
> opposition at the Inquiry...' [10]

The smoking gun

In May 1938, John wrote to Mr Wildgoose, who was collating the TB
inquiry evidence, with bad news about the latest statistics. The 1937 TB
statistics had now been released by the registrar general, much more
quickly than in previous years, perhaps in response to the political pressure.
'It is sad to notice that although the population of Wales decreased... the
number of deaths from Tuberculosis has increased.' Only three counties
came below the national average for England and Wales, with two counties
almost double the national average.

This was the smoking gun that Clem Davies needed. It was a direct
retort to the Ministry of Health's assurances that TB was going down in
Wales, despite not going down as fast as in England, and that there was no
need to worry. Now TB was going up! It showed the effect of the poverty in
Wales which had worsened during the years of high unemployment in the
1920s and 30s.

John's final submission of evidence to the TB inquiry ended:

> The ties that should bind us together in this great work are
> those of our nationality, and there is one injunction that we
> must not forget – it is 'Bear ye one another's burdens'.

John's work on TB in this era was helped by the publication of a book by
Scottish doctor and author Dr A.J. Cronin around the same time. Cronin
had worked for Tredegar's Medical Aid Society in the South Wales valleys,
where Nye Bevan was on its board, and wrote the bestselling novel
The Citadel in 1937. Cronin's book overtly criticized some doctors for
incompetence and seeking financial gain, and popularised the idea of an
organized health service free at the point of use. People understood the
concept as they had seen in the book – also made into a film in 1938 – how
poor health caused by poverty was not inevitable if people banded together.

Presidential address

The apogee of John's year as president of the National Conference of Friendly Societies was his address at the fiftieth annual national conference of the movement, held in Eastbourne on 22 September 1938.

Here, John could finally set out his overarching vision for a national health service to a huge audience representing the 12 million members, as well as a wide range of national press reporters.

It seems that he had learned from the rather controversial speech by George Lansbury about Hitler the previous year and this time no celebrity speaker was invited to the conference. This meant John's message could not be overshadowed in the national press.

So what did he say? Helpfully, in the days before the autocue, a booklet was printed out to accompany his speech.

John welcomed attendees and reminded them of the National Conference's achievements in recent decades:

> ... the National Conference has gone on from strength to strength in its participation in measures for social amelioration. Early in this century its representations to the Poor Law Commission were followed by consultations on the provision of the first Old Age Pensions in 1908. Collaboration in the preparation of the scheme for National Health Insurance in 1910 and 1911 was a landmark in our history. There ensued representations and pressure in 1917 and 1918 for co-ordinating the central services in a unified Ministry of Health, representations before the Royal Commission on National Health Insurance in 1925-1926 and, during the past year, the submission of testimony to the Committee of Inquiry as to anti-tuberculosis services in Wales...

As well as TB statistics, he also touched on cancer, which had seen a rise just as TB was falling, and generalised the point:

> It is the constant endeavour of our Societies to keep pace with changing conditions, and it behoves us to render all the assistance we can in any research which may assist in revealing the causation and possible remedial influences of and for such mortal diseases as these.

Two paragraphs are of particular note:

> The past year has been a somewhat arduous one for the officials of this Conference, especially in connection with the Tuberculosis Inquiry, but I think the efforts made in your behalf in that investigation will be well worth while and rebound to the advantage of the whole community, not only in Wales, but in England and Scotland too.

This is the inquiry John himself called for in his 1935 article about TB for the Royal Sanitary Institute journal and then campaigned for extensively. He modestly does not mention it was him behind this! When he says that it will rebound to the advantage of the whole community across the UK, what he hints at is that the Welsh TB group's policy request, which he provided the statistics for, may be about to be accepted. This was the request to form a unified national health service and provide better housing across the whole country, as the only way to eradicate TB, take the fight to the Giants and stop the cycle of reinfection. Also:

> The proposal of the British Medical Association for a General Medical Service for the Nation is another subject of current interest. It is proposed to include all persons within a £250 income limit and their dependants. These proposals are entitled to receive the careful and sympathetic as well as critical consideration of such an organization as this Conference in the interests of our members. They will certainly call for and receive scrutiny with regard to their financial elements and administration.

This is a unified national health service across the country, again stemming from the Welsh TB group's policy calls, which John did the statistics for himself. Despite it being John's own policy ask, he now talked about it here as if it was invented by the BMA. This is because in general in the health service there is a feeling of antipathy to anything NIH, as we saw earlier: not invented here. The BMA was also a notoriously prickly group at the time – after suggesting their 'General Medical Service for the Nation' in 1938 as John mentions in his speech, by 1948 the BMA were opposing Nye Bevan and encouraging doctors not to join the new NHS, which the BMA themselves had called for. Perhaps this was the reason for John's coyness about his own involvement in the original policy request for a national health service, as he needed to let the BMA feel ownership of it.

So, what did John and his Oddfellows colleagues think of his speech and the work on TB so far?

In the *Oddfellows Magazine*, John is quoted referring to the conference at an Oddfellows meeting in Sussex shortly afterwards:

> He was grateful for the comradeship shown to him on so many occasions in the great fight which has been waged against a frightful disease, and perhaps when the [TB inquiry] report was available they would appreciate that the fight was well worth while. (Applause.)[11]

On 5 November 1938 John received his own Meritorious Service Jewel, the highest award in the Oddfellows. John of course had the top jewel as he had led the national organisation of the friendly societies, and that is the ribbon my granny showed me in her attic when she first told me about John's work.

Bro. Toogood, past grand master, came to Community House, Newtown, to present it, with many tributes from Oddfellows leaders. He said that John's 'work would leave its mark in the Unity for all time... His wide knowledge and practical experience in almost every field of social service, together with this sympathetic consideration of every application for assistance, made him an ideal member of the [Investigation] Committee. His shrewd mind and legal training was of untold value in determining the various cases... [At the National Conference] he presided with great distinction. His presidential address on that occasion was a gem, full of vital information on Friendly Society work, the Social and Health services of the country, and urging a continuance of that spirit of fraternity and tolerance which had made the Friendly Society movement such a tower of strength.' [12]

The long wait

By the time John finished his year as president leading the friendly society movement nationally in 1938, it seems a grand total of nothing had happened as a result of the TB inquiry. Would anything happen? It was unclear.

On the one hand, the movers and shakers were all senior Liberals and radical socialists together and all based in the small town of Montgomery. Clem Davies, who was leading the TB inquiry, had taken over David Davies' seat as MP for Montgomeryshire when David chose to stand down, so they knew each other well. John and Clem also knew each other well, and John's son Edward was Clem's parliamentary agent for one election.

It turns out that Clem Davies was a highly influential politician who could fight very effectively for the cause of TB in Wales, if he could be persuaded to come on board. His grandson Christopher Clement-Davies recalls:

> One of the most striking aspects of Clem's time as a backbencher was the influence he exercised amongst leading political figures of the time. He was being drawn into meetings with Lloyd George, Baldwin, Ramsey MacDonald and John Simon before he had even made his maiden speech. This was part of a pattern that continued throughout his political career, a reflection, I believe, of the trust that many decision-makers placed in his judgment and intellect, as well as his integrity and straightforward sense of public duty. He said and did what he believed to be right, with little regard for the personal political consequences. For example, when Stanley Baldwin decided to step down as Tory leader and Prime Minister, in 1936, the first person he consulted was my grandfather, sitting on the lawn at Plas Dyffryn [in Meifod, Montgomeryshire] (which he described as 'a gem'). Attlee, Churchill, Eden and Macmillan were to consult him repeatedly during their premierships about critical decisions. Adlai Stevenson, twice Presidential candidate in the States in the 1950s, insisted on seeing Clem before anyone else whenever he came to London.[13]

Yet, on the other hand, David had also got into a public spat with his successor when David publicly challenged the Liberal Party's policy of appeasement leading up to the Second World War (which was in line with the other parties at the time).

Perhaps David had put his foot in it and Clem would retaliate by burying his TB inquiry report or watering it down a lot to gloss over the issues? As time went on without the report being issued, the possibility that the report would be a whitewash seemed more likely. Surely if it was felt urgent it would have come out more quickly?

John and David must have been feeling huge anxiety at this point. If the report was negative about the WNMA's work, it would be impossible to get further capital funding to update their hospital buildings and the organisation would eventually have to close. Their twenty-seven years' work designing and running the first ever national health service, the main focus of their careers, would have been for nothing.

While they were waiting for the outcome, John kept busy, with no less than four articles in the *Oddfellows Magazine* about TB appearing in January 1939.

Next, there was a huge personal setback for John. After several years of very hard work, he went into the Royal Free Hospital, then on Gray's Inn Road in London, for 'a severe operation' and stayed at least several weeks. Would he survive, and would he be able to continue to be involved with the TB fight, or would he have to retire? He was now 64 years old.

Thankfully a later update in the *Oddfellows Magazine* tells us that John himself had been well enough to write in and tell them that he was 'regaining strength at home... though not yet able to return to duty... I would appreciate it very much if you could say how much I have been touched by the messages I have received from all parts of the country and how glad I am that the good wishes of these esteemed Brethren are being realized.' The article concludes, 'Not more so, Bro. Tomley, than your brethren.'

Fortunately, John was soon contemplating his return to work and is 'looking forward to being able to soon resume active service... As it has been impossible to remain inactive he has busied himself with a supplement to the Tuberculosis Mortality Tables, and he has discovered some startling changes in the percentages.'[14]

Report and reactions

So, after years of John fighting for this inquiry, and providing the main piece of evidence in the form of his national TB statistics, what did the inquiry report say?

Surprisingly, parliamentary reports like this are not yet available online, so I went to the National Library of Wales to find it. It took up an entire book. The contents are well summarized in the many detailed press reports and long Parliamentary debate which followed.

One famous and much quoted paragraph read:

> There are houses with roses round the door, but inside they
> are not fit for people to die in, never mind live in.[15]

The immediate national press reaction to the publication of the TB inquiry report was astonishing. John would have been thinking that finally people were listening and willing to do something about not just healthcare services for TB in Wales, but the wider issues such as poverty, poor housing and poor sanitation that were the underlying causes.

These headlines are just some of those from the two huge folios that Clement Davies, who led the inquiry, collected in his personal papers, which were donated to the National Library of Wales. As I turned the pages from local press to national press, it was plain to see that the entire country was talking about it:

Daily Mirror: 'Britain's homes of death'

The Times: 'Tuberculosis in Wales – health services criticized – outspoken report'

Daily Express: 'Report lifts curtain on hell-holes of Britain – houses worse than Shanghai'

The Bulletin: 'Conditions of 'another world' seen in Wales'

Sheffield Telegraph and Daily Independent: 'Housing horrors in rural Wales'

The Evening Times, Glasgow: 'Welsh houses which baffle description – slashing indictment by health commissioners'

The *Mirror* explained:

> The report describes an inquiry carried out in Wales and Monmouth and unfolds, area by area, the story of insanitary, overcrowded homes and men and women struggling against ill-health.
>
> In it all there is one bright light – the women. The report pays tribute to the wives and mothers who struggle to live in heart-break houses… And every day they must fight against the same ravages of tuberculosis, 'y dicai' – the decline – the Welsh call it.
>
> In some districts, the Commissioners say, the medical officers are at fault, for their reports are 'so meagre as to be almost uninformative.'
>
> But the chief accusations are levelled against the local authorities.
>
> 'One medical officer,' the Commissioners say, 'told us that all sorts of wires are pulled to prevent this report becoming effective.'[16]

The *Daily Sketch* added:

> Housing conditions 'worse than the native quarter of Shanghai' are described by the Committee of Inquiry into the anti-tuberculosis service in Wales and Monmouth, whose report is issued by the Stationery Office this morning...
>
> Medical officers are in despair. They get houses condemned, but as the occupants die others move in, and it is impossible to disinfect the hovels. Housing plans are brought forward only to be ignored or shelved because they would mean higher rates.
>
> Sweeping changes in local government administration will follow if the recommendations of the report are accepted by the Ministry of Health...
>
> Whilst recognizing difficulties of administration the Commissioners are of the opinion that the authorities in these counties have fallen far short of their duties and of their obligations. We find that they have had insufficient regard for their powers or their duties or the advice which was tendered to them by their officers.
>
> In fact, they have failed in their trusteeship as guardians of the health and welfare of the people who elected them.[17]

By 16 March, the *Western Mail* was reporting that MPs were tabling parliamentary questions to the minister of health. In another article in the same paper, a medical officer had clearly been inspired by Cronin's novel *The Citadel*, where a doctor blows up a dangerous sewer that is causing infection as the local council has failed to act, referring to 'houses that should be blown up'.[18]

By 19 March, the furore was such that prompt and far-reaching action was already being discussed by the minister of health with the newspaper reporters, even before the House of Commons debate. Note that he was not proposing to supply any money to deal with these issues, and considered pulling down houses as more important as a first step than building new ones, raising the question of where the families were meant to live in the meantime. This appears incredibly out of touch.

> Mr Walter Elliot, Minister of Health... will tell the House that he is preparing an Official Circular to send to all local authorities in Wales, telling them that they must immediately:–

- Pull down rickety, filthy houses and hovels revealed as breeding grounds for disease.
- Provide more sanatorium treatment.
- Supply more free milk to counteract the effects of poverty.
- Undertake the building of more new houses.

In those places with specially bad housing conditions, and where the local council has failed to fulfil its responsibility in building new houses, an Inspector from the Ministry will be at once sent down to draw up a housing scheme for the district...

If any local council continues to neglect its duties in future after this warning it will be dismissed and its duties handed over to a State Commissioner [who] will be armed with dictatorial powers, and will be answerable only to the Ministry of Health for his actions.[19]

Discussion in Parliament

The official parliamentary record, Hansard, reported how John's TB statistics, the key piece of evidence in the inquiry, flowed through to the inquiry's final report and the discussion in Parliament.[20] Note how, thanks to John's statistics and influencing work, the discussion has moved on from just TB or even just health, to the question of poverty, housing, education – in fact the entirety of the issues which would be tackled in the Beveridge Report and by the consequent foundation of the welfare state.

And, to come neatly back round to where we started, one of the first things mentioned in the debate is a Blue Book (the inquiry report). Part of what had led to the dire state of health in Wales was the Treachery of the Blue Books 100 years earlier (mentioned mid debate as controversial yet still defended by the minister for health as a triumph at the end of this debate) and the history of institutionally racist oppression of the people of Wales – illustrating the direct connection between discrimination, poverty and health for oppressed people which continues today. During the debate there were constant references to race, with some blame cast on the Welsh race, and the minister for health showing a large number of colonial attitudes including stating that mispronouncing foreign place names was a good way to get on with foreigners like the Welsh.

In 1939, though, this Blue Book would ultimately be welcome for the people of Wales, for it heralded the foundation of the welfare state and NHS.

The discussion in Parliament was covered in the national and local press, who then picked up on the bigger picture and more of the different points made in the T.B. Inquiry Report as well as on housing conditions.

The *Daily Herald* reported the speech made by Welsh Labour MP Jim Griffiths:

> For three-quarters of an hour last night the House of Commons sat listening in silence as a Welsh miner pleaded for the rescue of his nation, not as an act of charity but as a measure of justice.
>
> Parliament was debating the recent horrific report of the committee which inquired into the anti-tuberculosis services in Wales and Monmouthshire, the report which scorned official language and talked of "hell holes" and such-like.
>
> Mr Lloyd George used to deliver speeches about the sunrise over the Welsh hills.
>
> Last night Mr James Griffiths made Parliament almost shudder as he painted the picture of the sun setting in the Welsh valleys.
>
> For the eleven years during which separate official figures have been issued for Wales, he said, the percentage of Welsh unemployment has never been under 20, and has risen to 38. The rough average meant that for 11 years a quarter of the population had been living on the "dole."
>
> FOOD THE FIRST LINE OF DEFENCE
>
> Wales was paying the penalty of tuberculosis because of its poverty. Great areas were "on the black list" for tuberculosis, maternal mortality and overcrowding.
>
> The first message of the report to the people of Wales, he said, was that the disease was man-made, and what man had done man could conquer. Therefore the people should rid themselves of the fatalism that paralysed action.
>
> "We are not facing a predestined plague," he flamed, "but a social problem, and we must work out our own salvation."
>
> For "malnutrition" in the report he substituted "semi-starvation," and passionately urged that the first line of defence against "T.B." was physical resistance, which meant good food and plenty of it.

His one criticism of the report was that the investigators had under-estimated the amount of malnutrition due to poverty and over-estimated the amount due to ignorance of food values.

"Give the mothers the money," he said, "and they will solve it."

The present allowance or the farm workers' wage made a cookery book a mockery.

FIRELESS SCHOOLS IN COAL COUNTRY
Children were languishing in Carmarthenshire due to lack of milk while millions of gallons were being sent away from that same county.

Coming to "the second line of defence against tuberculosis" – housing, he quoted the report: "Families herded together in dark, damp, dingy rooms." "Sagging roofs." "Haunts of germs." "Worse than Shanghai." "Hell holes."

One township in his own constituency had an historic castle on the hill, symbolical of the old Wales, "a beautiful and lovely place."

But below it were about 700 houses, and two years ago Ministry of Health officials reported that 400 of them should be demolished at once.

He spoke of the "hounds of economy..." "Little children trudge miles to school buildings that should have been pulled down 25 years ago, sitting on cold, hard benches with damp feet and wet clothes.

"There are no fires in a country where coal is running to waste and colliers are running to waste, too."

Wales was paying a terrible price because its economic life had been built on too narrow a basis. Wales had done nobly in building up an industrial nation, and now it was entitled to justice.

"If half the fortunes made in Wales and taken out of it by coal owners, royalty owners and landlords were available for us now we would sweep our country free from this disease in a few years."

The newspaper also reported that 'Mr Walter Elliot, Minister of Health, hinted at a forthcoming conference of local authorities in Wales which he would attend. He charged local authorities with responsibility, especially for housing.'[21]

Griffiths noted that the best defences against TB were healthy food, good housing, good heating and warm clothes and shoes, particularly for children. Now think about that in the context of the UK today, where health inequalities have increased because of austerity. The 1948 welfare state Jim Griffiths and Nye Bevan later helped to set up has been so eroded that even working people like nurses have to use food banks because they can't afford food. Social housing has been decimated, so that many people now live once more in overcrowded housing and disused shops, where COVID infection is rife and even TB is starting to spread again. Heating is too expensive for many people, and lack of heating causes illness. Parents get into thousands of pounds of debt from taking a £20 loan to buy school shoes for their children. We can now understand exactly why these were issues in the 1930s and why it was felt essential to act upon all the issues to tackle health inequalities.

Where did Nye Bevan fit into all of this? Jim Griffiths was friends with Bevan: they were both from South Wales and had been students together at the Central Labour College in London. Nye Bevan didn't speak in Parliament on this occasion. It could be because Jim was representing the same views from South Wales, or perhaps Nye hadn't been able to make it to this crucial debate. That week, Nye was busy taking part in a rebellion against the Labour Party. Stafford Cripps had set up a Popular Front with the Communist Party and others and Nye was supporting it. The very same evening as the Welsh TB inquiry debate, the Labour Party threatened Nye with expulsion if he didn't rejoin its ranks, and this was reported throughout the national press.

Had the TB inquiry report been left to run its course at this stage, with Walter Elliot as minister of health, it sounds like it may well have been buried under a long series of meetings and conferences with no real outcome.

Meanwhile, in April 1939, John presented an Oddfellows Meritorious Service Jewel to Bro. Hugh Hughes in Shrewsbury, who summarized the effect of John's efforts so far.

> Bro. Hughes, responding, thanked his old friend… He referred to Bro. Tomley's own great work for their Society, and said that Bro. Tomley had done more than any other man in Britain to focus attention of the ravages of tuberculosis. Referring to the recent Report on Tuberculosis in Wales, Bro. Hughes declared

> that had it not been for Bro. Tomley's efforts he doubted very
> much whether the report would ever have been prepared. In
> season and out of season, on the public platform and in the
> Press, Bro. Tomley had been like a voice in the wilderness,
> crying out against the bad housing, bad nutrition and ravages
> of tuberculosis. He was trying to awake the conscience of his
> fellow men and eventually he won them over and the fiery
> cross was carried to the House of Commons.[22]

An accompanying photo shows John looking rather tired and thin after his
operation, but back at work.

In May 1939, John attended the Oddfellows' Annual Moveable
Conference at Scarborough and the *Oddfellows Magazine* mentions him
16 times – a record even for him. He spoke about the need for TB patients
to be strongly encouraged by the Oddfellows to go to sanatoria rather than
infecting their families. Again, John's key role was foregrounded – Grand
Master Bro. Cundall said:

> It is my duty as the head of the Manchester Unity to pay
> tribute to the splendid pioneer work of our Bro. J.E. Tomley, a
> trustee of the Order, in the investigation of the tragic facts.[23]

Later in the same magazine, John's recent speech about TB in Wales to
the West Central Counties Group Conference was being serialised. The
magazine mentions how John was received by his audience and the national
leaders who attended:

> There was a thrilling moment in the conference when Bro. J.E.
> Tomley, P.P.G.M., of Montgomery, got up to speak. Almost
> simultaneously from the body of the hall Bro. J. B. Jones, a
> Llangollen delegate, stood up and sang 'Land of my Fathers,'
> and on this signal the whole assembly rose to its feet and
> joined in the refrain. It was a fitting ovation to an Oddfellow
> who has done such useful friendly society work both inside
> and outside his Order.

After explaining his years of work, John spoke of the TB inquiry outcome:

> I am proud and happy to tell you that practically the whole
> of the recommendations we submitted to Mr Clement Davies

and Dr Coutts are adopted by them in their report to the
Minister of Health...

John then discussed the various proposals: earlier diagnosis, with proper
engagement from doctors, systematic disinfection of affected houses,
clearing waiting lists of sanatorium treatment, and pursuing a 'village
settlement' for long-term recovery from TB. He continued:

> No time has been lost by the Memorial Association in their
> endeavour to carry out these recommendations. I have the
> privilege of serving on the Committee of the Association
> which has been appointed to choose the site for a new
> hospital to provide 250 patient beds and, as soon as a site
> has been provisionally chosen, to take steps to obtain the
> sanction of the contributing authorities and put the work in
> hand forthwith...[24]

In the October 1939 *Oddfellows Magazine*, John's speech about TB in Wales
to the West Central Counties Group Conference continued to be serialized,
this part returning to the subject of housing. Another subject also came up:

> ... the Committee report that there still exists in Wales a
> number of old schools, badly constructed, dark, ill ventilated,
> badly or insufficiently heated, with inadequate water supply,
> if any at all, primitive and most objectionable sanitary
> arrangements or insufficient sanitary accommodation, no
> facilities for feeding the children and poor or insufficient play
> grounds... They ask, 'Why should children be sacrificed and
> be called upon to suffer and possibly carry with them that
> suffering or the effects of it to the end of their days?'

And once again, a coordinated, national scope was essential: 'there is no
doubt that a scheme on a national instead of county basis possesses very
solid advantages.'[25]

Unfortunately, in the autumn of 1939, the whole of Britain suddenly had
other matters on its mind.

Chapter 7

'The Unknown Friend'
1940–1951

The TB inquiry reports and their follow-up had to be shelved in the first few years of the Second World War: Britain had enough to do to defend itself during Dunkirk, the Blitz, the Battle of Britain and the Battle of the North Atlantic.

Uncle John, J.D.K. Lloyd, recorded the view of Hitler by people in Montgomery, typified by Hannah Jones: 'They say this man abroad, this Heatley or whatever they call him, is a most covetous man – wanting everything. These men on the hill [the observer corps] was telling me he's not educated. The Gentlemen have got him in a corner: he's no scholar and they're asking him questions he can't answer!'[1]

John's son, Edward, became a glider pilot instructor, training hundreds of pilots for a planned glider invasion of France. On the eve of war, in 1939, he secretly eloped to Gretna Green to marry his sweetheart Jose.

Edward had been walking near the beach in Ynyslas in the late 1930s when he noticed a house on fire. He rushed over to help move the furniture out of the house and make sure everyone was safe. The fire was out of control and it burned to the ground. It had started in a chimney. He got talking to one of the girls who was on holiday there, Josephine Jessop, and then returned the next day to see how the family were. This was lucky as the first day Jose had just got back from a trip to London and Edward had thought she was a bit overdressed for the countryside and not his type. The next day she was in more relaxed clothes and he changed his mind. After a whirlwind courtship, Edward told his family he planned to marry Jose. They disagreed. The opposition wasn't so much from his father John but from Edward's sisters, who had hoped he would marry their friend. That was what we were told. Looking in the newspapers now though, I see that Edward had actually announced his engagement to someone else – so things had been quite far along with his sisters' friend and it is not surprising that they were angry with him for breaking off the engagement and upsetting her. Several years of falling out ensued.

In 1939, as the Second World War started, Edward volunteered for the air force. Before he left, he and Jose eloped to Gretna Green to get married, helped by Jose's Scottish friend, Scotty. Scotty organised things and let them use her address as their stated address on the marriage record.

Edward and Jose never told their families. They officially married at another wedding in Aberystwyth in 1942, followed by a reception at the George Borrow Hotel on the mountain road. Their wedding guests included the Bunners, the Lloyds (J.D.K.'s family), Mrs Vaughan Pryce, and Mrs Snow (Sydney, my other grandmother).

As they were already married, they were technically breaking the law by remarrying. Edward, who followed his father John into the family law firm, later became the registrar for births, marriages and deaths, and needed to have a spotless record to hold this position. So he and Jose had to keep it absolutely secret their whole lives that they had not exactly followed the law themselves. We only found out long after Edward had died, towards the end of Jose's life, when their son Christopher's mother-in-law and people from her village went on a tourist coach trip to Gretna Green. The marriage register happened to be open at the page showing Edward and Jose's marriage. Jose's children said to her that they had found the information online to spare her blushes that her in-laws and the whole of a neighbouring village now knew about her rebellious past.

After their second wedding, Jose accompanied Edward to live at air force bases around the Midlands. While Edward flew, Jose drove a NAAFI van taking refreshments around the base. Jose's younger brother, 18-year-old Peter, was not so lucky: he was captured by the Japanese and kept in a prisoner of war camp for several years.

By now John's wife Edith was ill with Huntington's disease and acting erratically. She was thought to have Parkinson's disease and dementia. At that time, there was no way to find out that this was a genetic disease, so the secret stayed hidden for at least another twenty years.

For John's business partner Sidney Pryce's family, the war was hard too. Sidney's son-in-law, Captain Jack Snow, was required for constant duty in the Battle of the Atlantic, as captain of the *Queen Mary*, the fastest ship in the world at the time, now converted as a huge troopship to transport US troops and other essentials from the USA. Jack's main job was to steer the ship at a fast pace without stopping to outrun the German U-boats lying in wait for them.

Sidney had retired and handed over his share in the solicitors firm to his son Vaughan Pryce. His grandson Angus remembers going up to Sidney's bedroom to see his grandad and counting out his pills for him, at age five.

As Angus later said, in those pre-NHS days clearly no one was bothered about whether Grandad had the right number of pills. Sidney was ill for some time and died in 1941.

Jack's wife, Sydney, was left behind in Montgomery looking after two boys, and heavily pregnant with twins at the start of the war in 1939. This must have been incredibly stressful. Four years later, in 1944, Sydney developed breast cancer and died when her youngest son, my dad, was four years old. Jack was given leave just before her death, so that the family could go on a final holiday at Borth on the Welsh coast, then had to quickly return to war. Sydney's brother Vaughan, John Tomley's younger business partner, and John's son-in-law, Uncle Jim Stewart, both stepped in to help out with the boys.

In 1939, novelist Geraint Goodwin became ill with TB again and spent some time in a sanatorium at Talgarth, on the edge of the Black Mountains, run by the Welsh National Memorial Association. His family moved to Montgomery, close to his home town of Newtown, where Geraint died in October 1941, at the age of 38. His daughter Myfanwy, at primary school with the Snow brothers in Montgomery who were her distant relatives, was about six years old. Her younger brother Hugh, born in 1939, was a toddler.

David Davies and his family were hard hit during the war too. In 1944, while launching a new X-ray mobile scanning unit at his flagship Sully Hospital, David volunteered to be the first patient to have a new type of routine chest scan. The scan revealed advanced cancer and he died in June 1944. David lived long enough to see the Beveridge Report, but not the securing of the full NHS which he had spent his life working towards, as well as donating much of his fortune.

Meanwhile David's son, David Michael, was killed in action during the war in September 1944, only three months after his father died. His own son, another David, became the third Lord Davies at the age of three. Little David now joined the Snow brothers and Myfanwy and Hugh Goodwin on the list of young orphans.

John's wartime activities

As with the First World War, John probably got involved in quite a lot that wasn't recorded in the papers due to wartime secrecy. It was likely that, just as in the First World War, he was involved in running coordinated hospital services, certainly at the start of the war, as he remained working as a local health commissioner throughout the war. This was the third national health service, after the WNMA and the First World War hospital services.

What we can say with certainty is this:

Clement Davies MP became an Oddfellow in early 1940 and John was his 'Right Supporter'. Clem's oldest son had just died from epilepsy, aged 24, so he needed friends around him. The ceremony took place in the hall in Shrewsbury where their historic TB inquiry had started, and Clement made a speech about the inquiry work, as reported in the *Oddfellows Magazine*:

> Bro. Davies mentioned that the report had been taken up in greater numbers by M.P.s than any report issued in recent times, and said that Member after Member had told him that they believed that things were exactly the same in their parts of the country... a reflection upon the way the country's local government had been administered...
>
> A great change was about to come over the land, declared Bro. Davies... When the war was over... there was a new life coming for us. The old order would be changed. It changed considerably after the last war, and it would change considerably when this war was over.
>
> Bro. J.E. Tomley... [said] that it was not only the Welsh flag which Bro. Davies had unfurled there, for he had also unfurled a flag in another battle against death and disease, it being in that hall that the opening sessions of his inquiry had taken place. That day, too, he had enrolled under another banner in the battle against death and disease by joining their Order.[2]

In May 1941, the grand master of the Oddfellows, Bro. O.B Meadmore, and Clement Davies visited Montgomery for the centenary of the Ark of Friendship Lodge in Montgomery, John's own lodge. This neatly brings us back to his father Robert's predictions in John's first meeting for the changes his generation would make, and hoping that John would live to see the centenary year. Despite his own poor health, John had managed it.[3]

In 1942, John was unwell again, and in 1943 at the Oddfellows' Annual Moveable Conference it was reported that he was retiring as a trustee due to failing health. As he had served for so long, he had been their most senior trustee for a number of years. The editor of the Oddfellows Magazine wrote a tribute:

> When Bro. Tomley reached the Board of Directors at the London A.M.C. he had behind him a record of work which made him the unknown friend of probably thousands who

had never known his personal handgrip and had never caught the gust of his enthusiastic animation. [He] was the essence of good fellowship; and behind it all there was the fact that he lived his life on a plane which made the best that his brethren could give him just the petals which fall from the flower... In everything he was just as thorough as a professional man should be, but the inherent charm of it all was that he was always struggling for the man or the child who could not struggle alone. Wales will never forget its Tomley...[4]

So, was that it? No, we know John by now – he would be back.

The Beveridge Report

Clem Davies lost a second child, his daughter Mary, in 1941. Despite this tragedy, he kept on with social reforms. John was no longer able to travel to London himself to participate in discussions, due to his previous illness, yet kept in touch with Clem regularly.

Clem's grandson Christopher Clement-Davies explains that Clem

found himself collaborating closely at this time with another leading Liberal thinker, William Beveridge. The two of them spent months discussing the social problems and solutions that were to be written up and published in the Beveridge Report in 1942, which became the basis of so many of the idealistic reforms of the postwar government... He threw his full weight behind the creation of the NHS.[5]

It is amazing how the links between events were so flimsy and could have been easily broken, so that the NHS and welfare state might never have been set up. Like in a relay race, each runner needed to successfully pass the baton on to the next person before they became unable to run any further. Tom Mills, the Oddfellows leader who had campaigned for TB sanatorium treatment back in 1906 before dying of TB himself the year after, was arguably the first runner. He passed the baton on to John, inspiring him to write his article on 'Pauperism and Its Antidote' in 1906, which was read by MPs including the newly elected David Davies and picked up by the *Manchester Guardian*.

John and David then became the next runners together for many years, inspired by Tom's story to pilot the first national health service for TB in Wales when they set up the WNMA in 1910, and then campaigning for the model of national health service organisation to be rolled out for other medical treatment and in England and Scotland too. They campaigned for the TB inquiry, yet David started to suffer from ill health in the late 1930s so John had to take the key role giving evidence at the start of the inquiry, as well as having collated much of the evidence. John then became too ill to work as well.

It was a stroke of luck that, by this time, Clem Davies had been inspired to take up the baton of the TB inquiry and could continue as the next runner. When Clem lost his first two children during the war, he might have given up. Yet he managed to keep going until the baton was firmly passed to the next runner, William Beveridge.

Once the Beveridge Report was out, meetings were held across the country by the Oddfellows and other groups. In Montgomeryshire in April 1943, Clement Davies naturally led the call to action, as the local MP and the author of the Welsh TB inquiry report which had led to Beveridge, supported by John. Shrewsbury Castle was an historic place to make such a declaration, with the Welsh knights clearly in English territory and ready to take over the rest of England as Merlin foretold in Arthurian legend. This time the Welsh would be taking over England with the roll-out of the national health service they had made possible. Not war, but an act of peace and solidarity which would be to everyone's benefit.

The *Western Mail* reported from the Oddfellows' meeting at Shrewsbury:

'I am calling for action on this report now,' said Mr Clement Davies, M.P., at Shrewsbury Castle, speaking on the Beveridge Report. 'Promises made during a war and not carried out during the war are soon forgotten when the war is over. We suffered that last time. I refuse to be a party to deceiving the boys who are fighting.'

... Sir William Beveridge had done all he had been asked to do by putting forward a scheme to deal with the evil of want. The suggestion was now made that it was too expensive. The truth was that they could not afford to do without it...

Mr C. B. Meadmore, Past Grand Master, said that with their record in the past the order wanted a place in the administration of any new scheme in substitution for the present approved societies. They had a record of 100 years of voluntary insurance.[6]

The *Oddfellows Magazine* also reported, picking up different points:

> Bro. Clement Davies went on to say that we could have afforded a Beveridge Report in 1936, and we could have afforded it 50 years ago... The Beveridge Report in itself would only close one small gap. There was another gap with which it did not deal – that of low wages. Things had been tackled in the wrong way in the past, and he warned people who said we could not afford the Beveridge scheme, and opposed it on the ground of finance, that however strong their opposition was going to be, they had lost before they had started. Health was not going to depend on a sixpence in income tax...

The friendly societies understandably had concerns about their own future:

> The Grand Master Bro. T. Little... briefly referred to the attitude which the friendly societies took towards the report. With many of the suggested provisions in the report they had no quarrel, and these were valuable contributions to the social security principles of the country. They were very much concerned with the Health Services of the country in the new scheme. The experience of many years made friendly society men the most qualified body of men on the subject of sickness. If changes were brought about which meant the taking over of friendly societies it would be a disaster.

John was able to lighten the tone – he 'humorously remarked that if they found any defects in the Beveridge Report one reason was that there was no representative of Wales sitting on the Beveridge Committee' – but the issue continued to be discussed. As Past Grand Master Bro. O.B. Meadmore said: 'The societies wanted a place in the administration of any scheme that might substitute the approved society system.'[7]

Whether John himself supported the idea of friendly societies implementing the Beveridge Report is not indicated. He had been a local health commissioner and on Ministry of Health committees long enough to realise perhaps that the government might well prefer to administer the scheme centrally, and if everyone would benefit because everyone would now be covered for health, unemployment, pensions and so on, then central administration was a price worth paying. Although it was less personalised, it was possible to ensure a minimum quality standard, and central administration was felt by the government to be more cost effective. Centralization would also enable the collection of statistics and other data to find out the current issues and tackle them. John and David Davies had run the WNMA, after all, for national TB treatment in Wales. That was how John collected his statistics and made the case that led to the TB inquiry and ultimately to the Beveridge Report.

By September 1943, the practicalities of the Beveridge Report's implementation were being discussed. The Western Mail reported on a speech by the new minister of health, Ernest Brown:

> Mr Brown addressed the annual meeting of the Association of Welsh Insurance Committees at the City-hall, Cardiff, presided over by Sir Ewen Maclean. He recalled that, prior to 1911, there was no State system for helping the sick worker unless he was eligible for help under the Poor Law. Many persons who then opposed National Health Insurance now pointed to the merits of its organisation, recognizing that it had proved its value, and was now an integral part of the national economy.

And now the importance of prevention which John and his colleagues had highlighted decades before was firmly in the frame:

> The new scheme must be aimed at prevention as well as cure. Sound health must be put first. It was not by accident that the Minister of Health was responsible for housing. There was the tremendously important principle of free choice of doctor. Added to that was the clinical freedom of the doctor in his treatment of the patient.

There was a reminder, too, from the insurance association's president Sir Ewen Maclean that

'A great beginning and a solid foundation for the all-in national service could be derived from the National Health Insurance Scheme' – again a foundation that the friendly societies had laid. John himself was at this meeting, and he is named at the end as having been elected the association's treasurer.[8]

But where was Clement Davies? Clem had suffered another tragedy – his son Geraint was killed in military training in 1942, the third of his children to be lost in wartime. He became deeply depressed and exhausted.

Later in 1943, John's ailing wife Edith retired as secretary of the nursing association. Sydney Snow held the event at her home, as one of the younger members, only months before she would develop cancer herself.

1945 – the moment of truth

In February 1945, the end of the Second World War was hopefully in sight and John and Clement Davies talked again about reconstruction and the implementation of the Beveridge Report, reported in the *Oddfellows Magazine*. Clem was back to campaigning for the social reforms he had helped prescribe in the Beveridge Report.

> A very important meeting was held at Welshpool, on 24th February (Montgomery District) under the auspices of the National Conference of Friendly Societies and the West Central Counties Group Conference... Bro. Davies referred to himself and Bro. Tomley being brought up in the atmosphere of Oddfellow homes; both their fathers being active and honoured members of their respective lodges...
>
> [Davies] finished up with these words, 'I pledge myself here and now to work inside and outside the House [of Commons] for the right of Friendly Societies to administer the new National Insurance.' He also counselled Bro. Stenson not to give up hope of him bringing Sir William Beveridge along with him for the third time, and promised to get him to come along probably in May, possibly to Shrewsbury...[9]

Meanwhile on the opposite page of the *Oddfellows Magazine*, one of the current directors, Bro. Reimann, was speaking at Grantham and summarised the trajectory so far for social progress:

> Remarking that it was over two years since the world had its interest aroused by the publication of the Beveridge Report, Bro. Reimann said its proposals were far reaching and widespread, but they were neither new nor revolutionary. It was evolution, the consummation of the revolution begun by Mr Lloyd George in 1911...
>
> 'It could not be otherwise,' he added, 'when we remember that the entire plan is but an extension of the present voluntary

and national schemes in which we have been associated for over 100 years.

'We cannot forget that during that long period the friendly societies have performed a service to their members and the nation which has resulted in bringing immeasurable relief in time of sickness and distress when there were no other measures except the Poor Law.'

Nye Bevan

The story of the NHS comes finally to Nye Bevan. As soon as the Second World War finished, an election was held. Despite supporting Churchill as a great military leader during the war, people didn't trust the Tories with post-war reconstruction: it was the Liberals and then Tories who had messed it up after the First World War, interspersed with Labour minority governments who could not practically get anything done. This time, people voted for a Labour landslide victory, with Clement Attlee as prime minister.

Attlee had been elected as a short-term Labour caretaker leader at the start of the war, after Labour leader George Lansbury was forced out due to his pacifism. Remember how Lansbury spoke at the same conference when John was elected as the president of the National Conference of Friendly Societies, and overshadowed the news of John's election? When war began, Labour formed a coalition government with the Tories, so Attlee became deputy prime minister, working closely alongside Churchill as PM and being involved with the Beveridge Report. Now, at the end of the war, people felt Attlee was trustworthy as he had been Churchill's second-in-command.

The Tories, including Churchill, were no longer in power. Neither were the Liberals, including William Beveridge and Clem Davies. Now the welfare and healthcare baton had been firmly passed from them to Attlee. And what would he do with it? The landslide election meant a stable, election-free period of five years from 1945 to 1950, allowing him to get on with the establishment of the NHS and welfare state.

At this time, Attlee looked around for the final person he needed to pass the baton to – a minister of health and housing. Aneurin Bevan was a passionate backbench MP who was a board member for a small friendly society, the Tredegar Medical Aid Society. Yet Nye had been a thorn in Attlee's side during the war, constantly criticizing the government. Could Nye turn out to be a hidden gem? Attlee thought so. By August 1945, Nye had suddenly been elevated from a backbench MP to minister of health and housing, and became the final runner in this story. The end of the story had already been foretold in the Beveridge Report and people had voted overwhelmingly for an NHS and welfare state. So much of the battle had been fought. Yet there was still the final round of negotiations, decisions and legislation which was required to put the NHS and welfare state into place. This was Nye's role.

Jim Griffiths, who spoke so passionately about the Welsh TB Inquiry report, became minister for national insurance in 1945 too. He worked closely with Bevan and Attlee to set up the NHS and welfare state.

I was surprised that, in this story, Nye enters the national stage so far towards the end. When Nye was later lauded as the founder of the NHS, many people were aggrieved as they had been working on it far longer than Nye – since before Nye was born, in many cases, like John's. John doesn't appear to have been aggrieved though. He would have seen that the left-wing radical socialism that he supported in the Liberal Party had now moved over into Labour, and it was Labour who were winning elections these days. And two Welshmen as ministers of health, housing and national insurance? Now there was an achievement John would have relished. Perhaps someone had listened to John's previous suggestion about the Beveridge Report, that it lacked the presence of people in Wales who had been most involved with setting up precursors to the NHS there.

Of the key witnesses in the TB inquiry, John was now no longer able to travel to London because of his health, and David Davies had died, so it was time for the new generation to take over. Nye may not have been directly involved in the WNMA's national health service for TB in Wales, but he had been on the board of the Tredegar Medical Aid Society, which organised a comprehensive health service for workers in one town in South Wales, and would have been a partner of the WNMA. The friendly societies employed the panel doctors who referred patients to the WNMA's TB sanatoria and other services. So Nye had seen things at the grassroots and knew how a health service should work.

Did John work directly with Nye as my granny had originally implied to me? There is one place they are definitely reported as working together, at University College Wales Aberystwyth, now known as Aberystwyth University. When John was an elected governor in the 1930s, Nye was an ex-officio one as an MP, and David Davies was president.[10] The governors would certainly have discussed health services extensively because the university's students had high rates of TB.

There is no other specific mention of John and Nye working together in newspapers and the *Oddfellows Magazine*, yet since they both spent a lot of time in South Wales and both worked in policy and influencing, it is fairly likely they crossed paths when working on health.

The Tredegar Medical Aid Society would likely have been sending patients to the TB sanatoria run by the WNMA, where John was on the board.

As John had been the president of the National Conference of Friendly Societies, and went there as an Oddfellows representative for many years, he may have met Nye representing the Tredegar Medical Aid Society, as one of hundreds of attendees. Many friendly societies sent their MPs and local councillors to the conference as it was the main political forum for the friendly societies and manged the relationship between the sector and government. John was also a speaker at the South Wales and Monmouthshire Oddfellows' annual conference. Nye as a local MP would probably have been invited there too.

John also had probably met Nye when he was working with Welsh MPs to get them on board for the TB Inquiry, although Nye did not attend the House of Commons debate in the end.

By 1945, Nye had the backing of Parliament and voters, thanks to the outcome of the TB inquiry report and the way this had changed hearts and minds across the UK. Suddenly people were willing to contribute to their own and others' welfare through increased taxes and National Insurance. Discussions started in earnest, led by the new minister of health and William Beveridge.

By now the direct role of the friendly societies was under threat but the situation remained fluid. And John remained an important presence at the Oddfellows' gatherings. Here's a report from one in Shrewsbury in October 1945:

> 'It will be a sorry day for our country when the spirit of the Friendly Society disappears from our midst. May your numbers grow and influence extend,' declared Alderman A. Bennett, mayor elect, when he welcomed the annual meeting of the West Central Group Conference...
>
> Greetings were read from Sir William Beveridge, who said he hoped to have the pleasure of addressing the Conference at some appropriate time...
>
> The chief business of the afternoon was an address from Bro. Tomley, 'Father' of the Conference, on the Joint

Committees' Report on Re-construction. He received a great ovation... Bro. Orton moved a vote of thanks to Bro. Tomley. Bro. Stenson, seconding, said Bro. Tomley was one of the few whose outlook and ideas did not get old and out-of-date with age.[11]

Around this time, the *British Medical Journal* (BMJ) also published praise of the WNMA as a model for Nye Bevan to look at:

The unification of the Welsh counties in this admirable tuberculosis scheme shows how the needs of a whole area can be planned without disproportionate regard for the natural but inconvenient loyalties of local areas. The Welsh Tuberculosis Scheme is indeed a model which should be studied widely by English counties and county boroughs.[12]

The debate over Friendly Society involvement continued in 1946 (John was again present):

Friendly Society representatives, principally members of the Manchester Unity, assembled at The Castle, Shrewsbury, on March 2nd, and were unanimous in their protests to the Government on the question of the exclusion of Friendly Societies as administrative units in the new scheme of National Insurance... The Mayor said that all right-thinking men realized that the Friendly Societies were the backbone of the country, and he did hope that a way would be found whereby the Government could make use of the great Friendly Societies of the country in the administration of the National Insurance Act...

Bro. H. E. Goodrich, Labour M.P. for North Hackney [said]... it had been necessary to remind the House of Commons that the National Health Insurance scheme would never have progressed but for the Friendly Societies...

'We have been asked to administer this scheme, and then when the machinery is working and he has got his offices going he will say, "Thank you very much, out you go, and I will come in,"' said Bro. Goodrich, amidst laughter. He went on to say that in his view the Friendly Societies were quite capable of handling the whole matter...[13]

But by October 1946, it was clear that the friendly societies would no longer be involved in the new state scheme:

> Alderman Charles W. Key, Parliamentary Secretary to the Ministry of Health, spoke on the Health Services Bill at the annual meeting of the Association of Welsh Insurance Committees [where John was still involved, now as treasurer] at Aberystwyth on Thursday.
>
> He said that the experience gained by insurance committees in administering medical benefit for a limited section [i.e. the friendly societies] had been most helpful in showing what kind of machine ought to be created to provide similar service for all. The success of the change over from the old scheme to the new would be largely in the hands of insurance committees and their officers, and the Government was relying on them to ensure a smooth transition.[14]

During this time of changeover to the new full NHS, the WNMA had regular meetings with the Ministry of Health staff and Clement Davies MP. A letter of 7 May 1948 in the WNMA records notes that a number of members waited upon the minister, Nye Bevan, as a deputation from the regional board. This may have included John, who remained active in Welsh national health committees at this time and was also still on the board of the WNMA and chair of its finance committee.

At these meetings, the WNMA also pushed for Wales to continue to be recognised as a unit and their TB services to continue to be run in a joined-up way. This was agreed by Nye Bevan.

In 1948, John was able to see the culmination of a lifetime of effort to change the world for the better. Finally, thanks in part to the TB inquiry which he had pushed for over so many long years, having provided the vital evidence through his national TB statistics and commentary, the world had indeed changed.

On 22 June 1948, Nye Bevan wrote to the Welsh National Memorial Association, whose services (including the sanatoria) were being transferred to the new full NHS, to thank them for their work. This letter is in the WNMA archives at the National Library of Wales.

> With the near approach of the day appointed for the introduction of the Government's new health measures and profoundly conscious of the manifold changes which

these involve I cannot but be mindful of the many excellent organizations whose life, as separate entities, draws to a close. Prominent among them is the unique fabric established in Wales over thirty years ago to deal with tuberculosis – prominent by reason of the uniform efficiency with which it has done its job; unique in its anticipation, so far as concerns broad outlines, of the pattern we have considered best for the future hospital service in general.

As the old order gives place to the new many cherished associations must unfortunately be dissolved, and I sympathise deeply with those who, at this time, must feel a sense of loss as their microcosm merges into the larger sphere. Good people such as these have deserved the nation's thanks for their magnificent endeavours, often in the face of formidable obstacles and despite restricting handicaps... It is common knowledge that, through the medium of the Association, sufferers of tuberculosis in Wales have been assured of treatment second to none and that your well equipped staffs and institutions have not only been a real bulwark against the advance of this dread disease, but have successfully carried the war into the enemy's camp. We look forward hopefully to greater conquests in the field of remedial and preventive medicine and do so with a confidence enhanced by the knowledge that your team of workers – in the council chamber, at the desk, in hospital, sanatorium, clinic and laboratory – have laid secure foundations and set an example of purposeful devotion for us all to emulate.

I trust that the spirit of the Welsh National Memorial Association will live on and infuse vigour into the wider service upon which, with a feeling of high adventure, we are about to enter.[15]

On the 25 June 1948, David Davies' sister Gwendolyn Davies wrote to the WNMA staff, following Nye Bevan's letter.

On July 5th 1948, the National Health Service Act comes into force. The change from the old order to the new, however desirable and necessary, involves the passing of the "Memorial" in its present form. As I said in 1946, this will inevitably cause feelings of sadness to those who recall with justifiable pride the faith and work of our pioneers and those who have followed on during the past 38 years. They blazed the trail for a Regional Hospital Scheme, which has now been adopted as a model for the new Health Service, with Wales as a distinct unit.

Whilst we cannot but deplore the passing of the Association as a separate entity, we must remember that the founders always envisaged – in fact the Charter provides – that, in time other diseases would be dealt with by the Movement inaugurated in 1910. That objective is about to be realised. The control not only of tuberculosis but of all Welsh Hospital services will vest in the Welsh Regional Hospital Board...

Commencing with a small sanatorium of 8 beds (the Penhesgyn Open Air Home, Anglesey), we have, by 1948, provided a regional specialist service of about 2,600 beds, linked with a network of 100 outpatient clinics, a mobile mass radiography unit, with a second unit in immediate prospect, an educational campaign, a tuberculosis laboratory and research centre, a Chair of Tuberculosis at the Welsh National School of Medicine, 50 distinguished specialists who participate actively and whose services, both in diagnosis and treatment, are freely called upon, a full-time medical staff of 70, a nursing staff of 580, and a domestic and outdoor staff at Institutions of 830.

Prominent in the wide field of health workers who can claim credit for what has been accomplished are the present members of the Association – this Board of Governors, the Council, the Central Committees, and the various House Committees of the individual Hospitals and Sanatoria.

It therefore affords considerable satisfaction to record that, in the setting up of the Welsh Regional Hospital Board and of the Management Committees, representation direct or indirect, has been given to the "Memorial". Nine members of that board and 69 members of those Committees are actively connected with our Association. This is evidence that it is recognised that their long and varied experience will be of inestimable value in a comprehensive health scheme.[16]

Not only could the working people John supported now have a doctor's appointment without fear of the cost, to ensure conditions such as TB were picked up early, but also the government was putting in place a wider welfare state which would tackle the root causes. A social security safety net would ensure a guaranteed minimum income, so that everyone had enough money for basic food and children's clothes and shoes so they could attend school; unemployment would be tackled through nationalised industries and creating additional public sector jobs; there would be centralised provision for decent homes in the form of a huge council housebuilding programme; improved facilities had been secured as a right in schools including sanitation, heating, free school milk and free school meals; free care would be given to people with disabilities; and a comprehensive public health programme would ensure that everyone was taught how to stay healthy and germ free, now that this was financially possible for all.

John started off aiming to slay one of the Beveridge Report's 'Five Giants', Disease. Yet, as is always the way of wicked problems in society, even today the giants are interconnected. Fight off one giant alone and the others come back stronger. The only way is to tackle them all at once. John learned this through fifty years of hard, bitter experience attempting to tackle TB in different ways. In the end, his TB statistics and the inquiry he pressed for led to a revolution in society which tamed all five giants.

Retirement

John retired as a local health commissioner, from the WNMA board, and from most of his other roles in 1948.[17] Finally, at 74 years old, war had ended and he had seen his vision of a full national health service and welfare state, which he had worked so hard to bring about, established as a reality for all of us. Now he could rest and enjoy time with his family. John's son Edward and his wife Jose had their first baby, Christopher, in 1947. John now had four grandchildren.

During this time, John also looked after his wife Edith, who was by then ill with what was thought to be Parkinson's disease and dementia, although, two decades later, it was realized to be Huntington's disease. She died in 1949, at the age of 72.

In November 1948, we hear what happened to the Oddfellows, who were coming to terms with no longer administering National Insurance (once again John was in attendance and given 'a very cordial reception').

> ... Bro. Mountford welcomed the National Insurance Scheme, which, he said, would provide for basic needs in sickness and other times of adversity, but looked at rightly, this should be

a stimulus to safeguard the personal standards which people had built up by voluntary supplementary insurance, and other forms of personal saving.

The Manchester Unity were the pioneers in schemes of social insurance, inasmuch as for 130 years they had helped the sick, the needy, and alleviated the distress of members and their widows. Since the inception of National Insurance members had found cause to complain regarding the delay in the payment of benefits, and they were now realising the great help they had received from Lodge secretaries when the administration of National Insurance was carried out through the Lodges...

Bro. George T. Orton, who spoke on 'The Challenge of To-day,' called for a greater degree of optimism and hope, to counter the fears and anxieties of the moment... Material success was of little avail, unless it was accompanied by friendship, love and truth, which were the very foundations of the Order... There was still ample and important work for them to do.'[18]

Ample and important work indeed. Many of the friendly societies transformed into cooperatives, pension funds, mutuals and building societies to help people on lower incomes save and afford mortgages. Societies like the Royal London and Scottish Friendly are still household names today – and the Oddfellows are still going strong, supporting many charities and local causes around the country.

A ringing endorsement

John had one last quirky surprise for us. In December 1949, the *Oddfellows Magazine* reported:

Bro. W Frank Stenson writes... '[On] the subject of bell-ringing, a short time ago I received some correspondence from Bro. Tomley (Montgomery) to the effect that there were a set of good hand bells at the Parish Church not being used; fifty years ago they were not silent, he used to ring them.

I passed this information of the Editor of the RINGING WORLD with a few observations with a view to re-kindling the old interest. I also quoted a few of Bro. Tomley's Activities and included a copy of the agenda from the annual meeting of the Conference last month, which included an item, 'Address by Brother Tomley, seventy years an Oddfellow,' and a suggestion that we might arrange an 'Oddfellow' peal in Montgomeryshire, to stimulate interest in the County.

The Editor of the RINGING WORLD seized on this suggestion, and further mentioned that the peal might be rung as a compliment to Bro. Tomley's lifetime of service to Oddfellowship...

As to the compliment, I would like to say that none was ever better merited... Bro. Tomley's most kindly and generous counsel and advice has been the guiding light of my Conference secretaryship, and I would like to acknowledge it here and thank him.'[19]

In September 1950, the National Conference of Friendly Societies took place in Scarborough and heard a message from John:

The President also took the opportunity at this stage to refer to the serious illness of Bro. J. E. Tomley, who was also a Past President of the Conference. He said that he had received a letter from his son, stating that his father often spoke of his friends in the Friendly Society Movement, and he sent his best wishes for the success of the Conference.[20]

In October, the bell-ringing event for John took place. John was ill at home after two seizures earlier in the year, and could not come to hear the bells himself, yet sent his daughter Esther to represent him and treat everyone to tea. John was very pleased to hear about it from Bro. Stenson who visited John afterwards. '[John] had looked forward to the peal for months, and talked about it for days. He also remembered that the Conference was meeting the following Saturday, and sent his good wishes to all present.'[21]

From the grave to the cradle

John died at home at The Hollies in Montgomery on 14 June 1951, aged 77. The NHS had pledged to look after people, as Churchill put it, 'from the cradle to the grave'. John and his wife Edith had been the first of our family to be cared for free of charge by the NHS at the end of their lives. Their granddaughter Susan, my mother, was born seven months later. She became the first in our family to be born under the NHS.

The Oddfellows Magazine printed John's obituary:

> Apart from his great work for the Manchester Unity, he was one of the best known public figures in Wales.
>
> As a legal man he was also a statistician. He compiled all the facts and evidence needed for Mr. Clement Davies' inquiry into the cause and effect of tuberculosis in Wales. He had been connected with National Health Insurance since 1912.
>
> Attending the first meeting of Montgomeryshire Insurance Committee after implementation of the Act, Bro. Tomley was elected clerk to the Committee and held that post until that body was succeeded by another committee under the recent National Insurance.
>
> Bro. Tomley became clerk to the new Executive Council and his intimate associations with national insurance since its inception lent added weight to his recommendations and suggestions. His interest in public health extended far beyond his statistical work for Mr. Clement Davies' inquiry into T.B.
>
> He was a governor and council member of the Welsh National Memorial Association for the Prevention and Treatment of Tuberculosis and, as such, did much to combat a disease particularly prevalent in Wales.[22]

John would continue to be mentioned in the *Oddfellows Magazine* for the next 15 years. In Clement Davies' obituary in 1962, there was one last reminiscence of his and John's work together:

> Two of the greatest thrills of his life, he said, were his initiation into his father's lodge...; and later, when he and Bro. Tomley, of whom Bro. Davies was fond of saying 'the solicitor made the Q.C.,' [i.e. John had made Clem what he was] were made to take a toast at a meeting of the West Central Counties' Group Conference in the Council Chamber of the Castle at Shrewsbury, the scene of many of his meetings whilst chairman of the Government committee of inquiry into the Anti-Tuberculosis Services of Wales and Monmouthshire.

Prior to the conference, Bro. Ben Davies, a deputy from Llangollen, and a very fine baritone singer, got up and sang the first verse of the Welsh National Anthem, 'Land of my Fathers,' which had been printed on the agenda; during the refrain the deputies rose to a man and Bro. Davies and Bro. Tomley were made to sit out the toast.[23]

We should perhaps all stand and toast Brothers Tomley and Davies, and Lord Davies too, for their tireless devotion to improving healthcare and living conditions, for fighting the Five Giants over so many decades, for without their work, we would not have the health service and the welfare state that all of our lives have been touched by.

Epilogue

After John

By the time of John's death, his oldest grandson David, Doris's son, was 16 years old. David was planning to follow in his father Jim Stewart's footsteps as a doctor. He was doing well at school and hoping to be the first in the Tomley family to attend university. John would have been proud.

Following John's death, David continued to study hard. He got into Cambridge University to study medicine and was a rising star. Meanwhile Edward and Jose had two more children, Sue in 1952 and Jane in 1957, bringing John's total grandchildren to six. Now that the country was recovering from the Second World War, the NHS was in place and rationing was over, it seemed that things were going well for the family.

Yet in 1960, tragedy struck. David was 25. He had graduated from Cambridge and was doing medical training in London. Although it seemed on the outside that David was doing well, he had started to struggle with his mental health. Over time, this became clear to his family too. David was particularly close to John's other daughter, his Aunt Esther. Esther developed cancer and was cared for by David's parents, Jim and Doris, at their home, White House, in Montgomery. In November 1960, Esther died. David committed suicide a few weeks later.

As recently described in former junior doctor Adam Kay's book, *This is Going to Hurt*, trainee and junior doctors have always been a high risk group for suicide. Tragically, this was just as much the case in David's time as it is today.[1]

David's parents were devastated by the loss of their son and Doris's sister Esther in such quick succession. Yet more was to come. At the time, it was a tragedy that John's daughter Esther had died early, yet his other children, Doris and Edward, still expected they would live to old age. They had no idea that they both had Huntington's disease and would pass the 'pirate's curse' down through their own families.

When I was at a Huntington's disease peer support conference a few years ago, the conversation in one group turned to how many family members had committed suicide in each person's family. While professionals do not like to mention it to us, we know perfectly well that there is a high suicide rate, probably the highest of any single group of people.

People in families affected by the disease see their parents making poor decisions, losing all their money, being abusive to their families and any remaining money being sucked up by huge care costs. They don't want that fate for their own children. Many people die in car accidents and the like in the early stages of Huntington's disease – if it is considered as a traffic accident, this is better for their families than suicide as it is easier to accept and means their families may be able to claim on their life insurance.

The exact suicide rate was never discussed until a peer-led film *Alive & Well*, was made in 2013. This stated the suicide rate to be around 25 per cent. At the conference I was at, each person around the table talked about the suicides or 'deaths in traffic accidents' in their family. Yet the link is still little known even to most of the doctors treating us, such as GP and general hospital doctors. It seemed to be kept quiet so as not to encourage more suicides. However, the effect is that most of us are not taken seriously when seeking mental health support and therefore do not get any support. It also means that the link between being people forced to pay high care costs and suicide, which has been going on since the 1970s, is only just being picked up now. So there was no clinical evidence for why people should not be asked to pay these huge care costs, especially when multiple generations of the same family are affected.

In our family, John's daughter Doris was the first to be diagnosed with Huntington's in the late 1960s, after developing symptoms over a few years. Although her mother had the same disease, it was not well known in those days. Doris's husband Jim would not have learned about it in medical school. Genetic testing was not available, so families usually had to wait for at least two generations to develop symptoms before Huntington's disease could be confirmed.

Huntington's is one of the worst genetic diseases because it is carried on a dominant gene. Most genetic diseases are recessive genes, so only appear in one in four children – a quarter of the family would therefore die. With Huntington's, the odds are one in two children – half the family would die. Which half could not, of course, be predicted in those days. Many young people in Huntington's disease families have a normal clumsy moment such as dropping a cup and convince themselves they are developing symptoms. The disease can strike at any age – when I was diagnosed with the gene at age 23, I was told for that particular gene repeat length, I could get Huntington's at any age from 20 to 70. As I was already over 20, this has meant no respite period when I could be confident about my health. Over time, this constant trauma about when are you going to die exactly becomes very tiring.

People with Huntington's have been hugely discriminated against. We were the first to be banned from emigrating to America, and among the first to go to the gas chambers in Nazi Germany, hated even more than Jewish people or Black people. Up until the 1930s, people were thought to have Huntington's disease as a punishment for practising witchcraft in the family.

In the NHS, Huntington's was thought to be a mental health issue and people were put into mental hospitals where their physical neurological symptoms were not understood or treated due to a lack of understanding about the disease. This in fact is what happened later to John's daughter Doris, who was a patient at Shelton mental hospital in Shrewsbury from 1971 until her death in 1972.

Despite the set-up of the NHS, mental health was still very underfunded, and what we would consider inappropriate today, such as requiring people to live long term in institutions rather than at home, was still the norm as late as the 1960s and 70s. In 1968, Shelton mental hospital had also been the scene of a deadly fire, one of the worst hospital fires in NHS history.[2] [3]

John's son Edward, my granddad, was very upset by his sister Doris being in Shelton, especially as he was at risk of Huntington's too and was diagnosed himself a few years later, in the mid-1970s. Shelton was in a former Victorian asylum building where, in the past, people with the worst mental health conditions from the surrounding workhouses such as the Forden workhouse would have been sent. Like many former workhouse buildings around the country which transferred to the NHS in 1948, the facility was now run by NHS doctors and nurses who were as kind and caring as possible, and of course patients were no longer forced to work. Yet most people still looked on the workhouse buildings with trepidation and didn't want to go there. After the Shelton fire, there was a further reason to be fearful.

Edward's wife Jose, my granny, then asked my mum and dad to move from near London, where my mum had a good job at a solicitor's firm and was slated to become a partner, back to mid Wales to help look after Edward. As Edward did not want to go to Shelton, home care was the only option. During the 1970s, families like mine fought for the right for their loved ones to be looked after at home. This was eventually won, thanks mainly to the national outcry after the Shelton fire. Long-term care for most people transferred from the old workhouse hospitals run by the NHS to home care run by the new social services departments being set up in local authorities. Yet, due to political wrangling, the NHS did not transfer a lot of the budget, but held on to it.

Starved of funding, local authorities had to start charging people. Quality suffered, and new quality standards were brought in. But this just made care more expensive for people who were self-paying. Many people started losing their savings, and if they went into a care home, their home would be sold to pay for the care too. Their children inherited nothing and had to start from scratch in life, resulting in poverty and stress. For children and young people whose parents were dying early, this was a triple tragedy. Suicide became the only way out of the cycle, and it still is today.

For families with genetic diseases like Huntington's disease, each generation keeps going through the same cycle, with a knock-on effect on the whole family. Each time a family member died of Huntington's we breathed a collective sigh of relief that now we could go to the normal clothes shops instead of just charity shops. Now we could go to a supermarket and buy what we fancied eating. Now we could go for a meal out, or on holiday. But then the next member became ill and the whole thing started again. Now it's my turn next.

My mum got ill when I was a student and lost her business, home and savings, the lack of funds being a big worry for another reason too. I had been tested for Huntington's at age 23 and found out I had the gene so would definitely develop the disease sooner or later. Without any family savings to fall back on, the situation for my own future care had changed a lot. My granny Jose had always assured me that she was saving up as much as possible so that things would be all right for her grandchildren. I had to readjust to the fact that her savings had been lost by my mum, and I was now going to be reliant on just the state safety net. I might not be able to afford to be cared for at home, yet specialist young adult care home fees were astronomical too. The way care costs work is designed for older people with shorter illnesses, grown-up children and people with pension income. The amount people are allowed to keep makes no provision for their children's future costs as people are assumed not to have dependent children. It also makes no allowance for the fact that many people below the pension age do not have pensions, and therefore need income in future for their own living costs and essentials such as home maintenance.

Even more urgently, a new type of IVF treatment could enable me to have a baby without passing on Huntington's disease. IVF costs a lot of money too. Without savings it could take me longer to have a baby, meaning the baby would be younger when I got Huntington's, causing the child a lot more complications in their life and possibly losing their home due to my care costs. So the pressure was on to save up and have IVF as soon as possible.

My mum hadn't wanted to be tested, another issue with her decision-making earlier in her illness, so if I wanted the new IVF treatment that could let me have a baby without passing on Huntington's, the NHS required that I had to be tested myself first, and then had to keep my result secret to only two close friends. Imagine you found out you are going to die. Now imagine you can't tell anyone in your family, or your employer. That was what I was asked to do, at age 23, while also organising my mum's care and then fighting the loss of her business and home, working full time and saving up for a mortgage and IVF.

Doctors also advised me that I should not tell my employer as I was likely to be discriminated against. After a week off 'on holiday' after my diagnosis, I had to go back to my colleagues at work and tell them what a nice time I had. 'What did you do?' one of my managers asked. 'Oh not much, just pottered around,' I said. I could not tell them the truth, that I had found out I was going to die early and had been lying in bed for a week crying. I could not take any additional sick leave or be supported by my employer.

It was like living a secret double life, but the opposite of Superman. Death Girl perhaps? My secret double life was far worse than my apparent life of career success and carefree twenty-something professionals partying in London. No mental health support was available as this was part of an experimental period to find out whether people in my situation needed it or not. We were only followed up for a few years, so it was concluded we didn't.

Of course, with the benefit of hindsight, many of the multiple long-term conditions I now have are stress and trauma related and likely originate from this time and the lack of NHS support. My other medical conditions have cost the NHS more to treat than the original support would have done. In the past, there was no treatment available for trauma, yet even talking to someone would have helped. Now trauma treatment is available in the form of eye movement desensitisation and reprocessing (EMDR), which has been shown to be effective. It is not much different in cost to other mental health treatments, but was until recently not available on the NHS so was limited to people who can pay. I could not understand why this opportunity to stop so many mental and physical health issues at source in a cost-effective way was not being rolled out to everyone who needs it. Fortunately, some NHS staff are now being trained by Health Education England in a programme that started in 2021, although the treatment is currently only available to NHS staff who have had trauma at work. Perhaps in another ten years a few of us facing early death might actually get to try this out.

In 2007, we managed to move to a family-sized home and started to do it up. Now we had space for a baby. In 2009, we started IVF and in 2011 we finally had a baby. Thanks to NHS research, my daughter was born with a low risk of Huntington's disease and all the previous struggle had been worthwhile.

Meanwhile, my brother and my other cousins found out that they are unlikely to have Huntington's. For the generation of John Tomley's children, the dice of a 50:50 chance each time fell badly, so that two out of three of his children had Huntington's disease. Two generations on, among his great-grandchildren, I am the only one to have the gene and hopefully the last in our family.

Of course, if it hadn't been for John Tomley's pioneering work in studying TB and pushing for wider healthcare and welfare support, we might not have had the NHS at all, and every form of state-supported healthcare, however hard won, helps real families in real situations like ours. It is an unfortunate irony that his own wife was carrying a genetic disease which would affect his descendants in this way – but we must always be grateful that he sowed the seeds for hope in the future.

The fight against the Five Giants continues, and there are certainly lessons we can continue to learn from John's work – proper holistic thinking around health and social care, tackling housing and poverty, focusing on prevention as much as cure, gathering better data, showing compassion for the disadvantaged, and hounding government when required. Those are the golden keys he gave us.

Afterword

The Five Giants Today

So how does the fight against the Five Giants look today, for everyone across the UK?

We have the upper hand in health now, as the centralised organisation and resourcing of the NHS has led to many health breakthroughs. People having fatal medical conditions below the age of 65 is now, thankfully, much rarer.

Yet there are still a number of us in this situation, and those of us who are tend to be in areas which are historically Cinderella services such as genetic diseases, autoimmune conditions, the hard to diagnose and the undiagnosed – including the stubbornly large group of working-age women who are continually told by male doctors that there is nothing wrong with them, until they die of it. Awkwardly, the death statistics tend to put us all down as influenza and pneumonia, or a vague 'signs and symptoms' category, which are the final things that kill us off, rather than the actual underlying cause.

Our diseases are not that rare either – for example Huntington's disease, if anyone actually bothered collecting the real death statistics so we could be certain, in a way that John Tomley might have done. Huntington's affects 32,000 people who are at risk. Most people die about age 50, so this means about 640 deaths per year in the UK – although we know the true number is understated because of the pattern usually not being noticed in families until the second generation, the reluctance of families to come forward due to stigma associated with the disease, and the lack of track and trace for families. So, let's say the real figure is 200 more, 840 deaths per year. This is similar to cervical cancer, 853 deaths per year in the UK. We all know what huge resources are put in to finding and treating cervical cancer, so why is the situation so different for Huntington's? The lack of death statistics seems to be the key issue here.

Some of the advances which were made when the welfare state was started, and since, have been eroded over time. When people ask the government to spend more on one thing, another thing has to be cut to pay for it, and sometimes it is the wrong things. I am thinking particularly of the slow slide into overwhelming debt due to a mum on universal credit being unable to afford to buy their child new school shoes, and having to resort to a payday lender for £20, and this debt spiralling to hundreds or even thousands of pounds, causing them bankruptcy. I am thinking of people with disabilities, especially those of us with fatal diseases, having to cope with a terrible diagnosis and then be treated as worthless benefits scroungers, expected to work until we pretty much drop dead. I am thinking of the majority of young people now, unable to access affordable housing due to no new council housing being built, and even those who are 'well off' graduates ending up cash-strapped due to a huge student debt. The very families found to be most prone to TB and other disease in the 1930s are now being forced into overcrowding again, and the disease has been resurging. I am thinking of the huge cuts to the public health budget, a key plank in prevention. The cuts to other preventative and self-management services, especially in the voluntary sector.

Many leaders and senior managers already know this across the NHS, other public sector bodies and the charity sector. (I recommend Sir David Haslam's recent book *Side Effects. How our healthcare lost its way, and how we fix it*, which was published in 2022.)

Radical administration

John Tomley's approach was to get radical things done but by subtle means. He chose to tread a very pragmatic middle line between outright illegal rebellion, which his local friends the Farmer sisters chose when they were active in the suffragette movement, and the stuffy Victorian administration which was holding back efforts to tackle inequalities in health and social care.

History shows that both John's way of doing things, and the suffragettes' protest way of doing things, are necessary for change: first people protest, and then leaders in positions of responsibility can affect radical administrative change. Both groups need to work together to coordinate movements. Any kind of government body, including local government and the NHS, is a terrible tool for this, as those bodies must stay non-political. That is why the charity sector is so important today: like the friendly societies of the past, charities can bring together the people affected at the grassroots, the protestors and the administrative and political leaders and communicate effectively between the groups, while also inputting highly effective independent policy advice on what works.

Charities also have a history of helping the NHS try out new things, because it is often too complicated for large NHS organisations to try lots of different things. This means the cycle of trying new pilot services, measuring impact and replicating successful pilots to other areas can happen a lot quicker with the charity sector involved.

For this to continue in future, two changes are needed. Currently the action of civil society is being strangled by lack of finance and gagged politically at the same time, so is unable to function as a mediating force in society. First, the charity sector has had a huge amount of funding cut during austerity which needs to be replaced, and second, the recent law which reduced the ability of charities to work on political issues needs to be rescinded urgently. The rise in inequality on all measures is a clear indication of the outcome if we do not achieve this.

Systems thinking

The original architects of the NHS, including John Tomley, used what we now call systems thinking, although they didn't call it that in those days. It was just something that came with many years' experience of dealing with individual people who were patients in the pre-NHS health and social care services. Now health and social care services are huge and very siloed, which means many different organizations and their staff deal with each of a person's different issues, and very few staff can develop an overall holistic view of what determines health and how we can best change the system to improve people's health outcomes.

When the NHS was first set up, this was at the same time as the rest of the welfare state. As well as health services, other key areas of need were tackled at the same time, including poverty, unemployment, poor housing, poor education, trauma, disability, discrimination, crime. The experienced people setting up the NHS had themselves managed frontline services and therefore had an innate understanding of what are now called the social determinants of health: in other words, the Five Giants. In the last few years, public health statistics work has led to the much-heralded rediscovery of what the founders of the NHS already knew: over 50 per cent of health outcomes are not determined by NHS service provision at all, but by the other social determinants of health. For example, a person living in poverty may not be able to afford to buy healthy food; they may be more likely to live near a main road or have black mould in their home, so that their children are more likely to develop asthma; and they may be working long hours or traumatised by having been a victim of the high level of crime in their area, meaning they are more stressed and therefore more likely to develop physical health conditions.

Once a person has one issue, more issues are likely to happen and reverberate down the generations of a family. For example, a person may develop a disability and become unable to work. They become unemployed as a result, losing their income. They can't pay their rent or mortgage so lose their home. Their remaining savings are taken to pay for professional carers, because the state system is set up thinking about retired people with no dependents, not younger people with children to support. Their child sees the state care provided is very paltry, so after they leave school they stay with their parent as a family carer and do not go to university. The child then has fewer employment options so is on a lower income. The child doesn't have any savings inherited from their parent, so can't put together a deposit to buy their own home. The child has to pay much more in rent over their lifetime than buying their home would have cost. Any further disability or illness in the family then means they are vulnerable to losing their own home in turn and the cycle starting again.

When we think about it like this, from an individual person's point of view, this is just common sense. We all know if we were in that situation what would happen to us. So why is it so difficult for us to turn this insight the other way around and use it to develop more effective health and social care interventions which start at the beginning of people's journeys, with prevention of the underlying causes?

One answer is politics, both big P politics in Parliament and small p internal politics in NHS organizations. In NHS organisations, every manager needs to fight for funding for their local area or their department. So they have to get elbows out to fight off their funds being cut and continue to keep their staff and so serve their patients. Cutting hospital budgets is always a huge political hot potato, so MPs made sure during austerity that the hospital budgets were ring fenced from cuts.

This meant the large cuts during austerity were even more concentrated elsewhere, on prevention, self-management and home care. Yet all these areas are cheaper than hospitals, so people who are not getting these services any more end up with their conditions worsening and turning up at A&E. A&E attendance goes up. MPs say 'We need more money for A&E!' More money gets diverted from prevention, self-management and home care to fund A&E. So even fewer people get those services and even more turn up to A&E, in a vicious circle of spiralling costs per person and worsening services.

Older people needing home care can't be discharged from hospital because there is a shortage of home carers and minimal local authority budget to pay them, so hospital ward beds are full and there is no room for people to be transferred from A&E. Newspapers say that people are waiting on trolleys in corridors in A&E, so people are kept outside in ambulances to wait instead. The ambulances are then full and can't go out to the next patient. That patient who might before have waited 20 minutes for an ambulance now has to wait 10 hours. If it was urgent enough to call an ambulance in the first place, chances are that some people will die before the ambulance arrives. The newspapers have a field day.

To turn back this vicious circle, we need to unscrew the crank on the system and start pumping things the other way:

- Too many people in A&E?
  Step up prevention, self-management and home care provision instead, to divert people away from A&E before they reach the door, and improve the flow through the hospital once they are there.

- Don't want to cut hospital budgets?
  Then reinstate the level of separate budgets there used to be for prevention, self-management and home care provision, pre austerity. These were never overly generous, yet at least took the pressure off A&E somewhat. A larger investment than in the past could pay dividends here, as prevention, self-management and home care are all cheaper than A&E.

- Ageing population?
  All health and social care budgets need to increase according to the additional headcount, so that health and social care services are not desperate for funding and fighting each other to get sufficient funding. While digital health may save money in some areas, this is offset by the fact that, thanks to NHS success in saving lives, more conditions are now treatable longer term, and more people survive other illnesses to eventually die from dementia which is more costly to care for, so average lifetime cost per patient has gone up too.

It's just common sense if we all step off our own little hamster wheels we are running on and take time to look at the bigger picture together.

Systems thinking has always been used informally by many people, especially people who have many years of experience in delivering health and social care frontline services. As a formal management theory, it was mainly developed from the 1970s onwards and originally was applied to engineering processes. Over time, people realized it could be applied to other types of systems too, including complex health and social care systems.

We can then look to find points of leverage where the application of a small amount of resources leads to a substantial improvement. For example, health prevention is nearly always much cheaper than providing any kind of cure. If we can stop the illness beginning in the first place, it is so much better for the patient too.

Big data

The original architects of the NHS, including John Tomley, also used what we now call big data. This means gathering lots of data in order to have reliable evidence for making good decisions about health. In John's case, he was compiling the first national statistics for a disease, in this case tuberculosis. As well as the basic numbers, John also analysed the statistics in various ways in order to find underlying trends. He compared statistics from one place with another, and across years. He used graphs and maps to show prevalence of TB. He looked at whether interventions made any difference to TB rates.

For example, John found Wales had more TB than England. Then within Wales, west Wales had more incidence of TB than east and south Wales. West Wales was more rural so you would think people would be more spread out and less likely to give each other TB. Yet John worked out that things were more complex than this.

First, people in rural areas often had little or no access to a doctor due to distance, not being able to afford to pay a doctor and the first national health insurance only covering employed people and not retired people, women, children or sick people of working age. Clearly, not being able to see the doctor at all is a key reason people would have worse health. Here, John's statistics made the case that the fragmented system of healthcare needed to be replaced by a comprehensive universal national health service, covering everyone from cradle to grave, regardless of ability to pay.

Next, people in the most rural communities tended to be much poorer than people in the industrial areas as there were fewer jobs, and more sick people who had come home from the industrial areas due to their sickness.

Poverty is the biggest social determinant of health. People on the lowest incomes could not afford to live in homes with more than one bedroom. The TB inquiry found many homes where the sole bedroom had a double bed below and another bed on wooden planks directly above – like a big bunk bed. Often eight people or more might sleep together in these beds. If all the family members, including the older and sicker ones, slept together in these beds, then they were close enough to all their family members to breathe out TB germs and give them the disease over time. People on the lowest incomes also faced a number of other issues such as being more susceptible to disease because of poor diet, lack of utilities such as heating, water and sewerage, lack of warm clothes and shoes and so on. Here, John's statistics made the case for tackling the other social determinants of health, via the welfare state. If everyone had a minimum standard of housing to live in and a minimum income which was enough to buy basic food, utilities, clothes, shoes and so on, then everyone's health would improve and we would save money as a society because we wouldn't constantly be reinfecting each other with preventable diseases. People of working age would be able to earn more money, and employers would benefit from fewer sick days in their workforce.

What does big data mean now for the NHS and welfare state and why is it important today?

In *The Patient Will See You Now: The Future of Medicine is in Your Hands* (2016), Eric Topol, a doctor, surveys the different types of big data that are now available on a scale never before seen:

- Data that is already on databases about people, from Facebook to clinical databases. This could provide enormous opportunities to explore the social determinants of health, find out what works in terms of interventions, and act accordingly.
- Data that can be collected through technology such as smartphones, for example diagnostic medical tests conducted by the smartphone itself or an attachment, e.g. to take a fingerprick blood sample and analyse it on the spot. People could also enter their own symptoms in a questionnaire and get a diagnosis, rather than having to see a doctor.
- Genetic data – now the cost of sequencing a genome has hugely reduced to about USD $1,500, how long will it be until everyone automatically has their genome screened to identify all genetic diseases?

Topol explains that, of course, using big data for diagnosis is not going to replace the need for doctors in general. But technology might mean that doctors can be freed up to give more personal support.

Key policy asks

Here is a list of key policy asks for today, based on what we have learned from John Tomley's efforts and the original foundation of the NHS and wider welfare state. This of course includes a statistical one.

In formulating these through conversations with senior politicians, civil servants and health and social care staff, the dilemma that kept coming up was whether to tweak the system, which is what was done before the foundation of the NHS and welfare state, or change it entirely to fill the gaps and once more have a comprehensive safety net that covers everyone from cradle to grave, which is what was achieved by John's statistics and the resulting Beveridge Report. Tweaks are much easier to achieve. Long-term change takes time. Time is the one thing that those of us who are going to die early don't have, so I have started with a tweak for my own situation and then suggested long-term changes to benefit everyone.

1. Die Early For Free

This is a policy tweak which would be relatively simple and low cost: those of us aged under 65 who are going to die early should have our savings disregarded when it comes to care costs.

When we are told we are going to die early, that is a huge shock. The doctor doesn't at the same time tell you 'By the way, you will lose all your savings' as that would be too cruel a shock on the same day. So we think, 'Ah well, I am completely screwed on the health front but at least I have savings to live on and to pay my child's living costs, and hopefully if there is enough to pay for my funeral then my child may be able to inherit enough money to start them off in life even though they have been orphaned and I am no longer there to look after them. And maybe we might go on a few trips together for my bucket list before I die, so they have some nice photos to remember me by.'

For cancer, this is correct. Yet for other diseases, such as Huntington's disease, this is completely wrong. Our savings will be lost to care costs so there is no chance of a bucket list. Maybe you can afford a bucket, that's all.

The unfairness of care costs for people of all ages has already been recognised by the government's own Dilnot Report in 2011, over a decade ago. This led to agreed reforms including a care costs cap, but these have been delayed in England for many years. Meanwhile, Wales has introduced a much lower care costs cap of £5,000 per year for everyone. Scotland has also introduced some types of free social care. Yet without the tax contribution from the UK parliament to pay for these, care is effectively still being rationed at the point of delivery.

So how much would it cost to Die Early For Free? In the spirit of John Tomley, we can work this out.

The total number of deaths in England and Wales in 2021 was 586,000. Of these, the vast majority of deaths were over age 65. Wales and Scotland already have much more generous care caps than were proposed for England, so we only need to consider England. The total number of deaths per year of people age 20–65 in England, apart from cancer (where care is already funded), Covid-19 (due to the pandemic that year), accidents, suicide and pregnancy was 33,000.[1] These are the deaths that may involve care which is currently unfunded. Some of these deaths will be immediate, for example from a heart attack, and will not involve any need for care. This means the figures quoted below are the maximum, and would probably be somewhat lower in practice.

According to the Office for National Statistics' Wealth and Assets Survey 2022, half of adults have less than £12,500 in savings so will not be affected by the care costs cap – the state already pays for all their care. (This is why we need longer-term reform to make sure everyone facing early death has a liveable household income.) So, the maximum number of deaths that might involve unfunded care costs is halved to 16,500.

£58,500 is the 75th percentile of savings held by all adults, including retired people. People facing early death have had less time to save up than retired people, and younger generations have also faced much higher costs for rent, mortgages and childcare. So, let's assume that people facing early death have half the savings and our 75th percentile is therefore £29,250.

So we estimate that for the half of early deaths where people face unfunded care costs, the 16,500 people, each person has average savings of £29,250. With people able to keep £14,250 of their savings, an average person will therefore contribute £15,000 to their care costs over their lifetime.

The total cost of Die Early For Free is therefore £248m per year. The UK had total income tax receipts of £348bn in 2020-21, so the additional tax needed would be 0.07 per cent of this total.

With a main income tax rate of 20 per cent at the moment, this means income tax would need to increase to 20.014 per cent, a vanishingly small amount to correct the huge current injustice for those of us faced with the double whammy of early death and care costs. Alternatively, the policy could be very easily funded by increasing the higher rate of income tax or corporation tax back to their historic levels.

2. A new early death inquiry

As we've already seen through John's story, the original TB inquiry looked into the causes of early death due to TB, which at the time was the main preventable cause of early death. Now TB has been mostly eradicated, and early death below age 65 is relatively rare. Yet there are many other preventable causes of early death which still exist today, killing thousands of people each year. These causes have not been looked at in the round for a long time. Now, on the 75th anniversary of the NHS and welfare state, the time has come to once again look at early death in detail, in order to take coordinated action against preventable early death.

As with the TB inquiry, we know that for every death, the same causes were leading to many other people having disabilities, as well as the stress caused by the whole family falling into poverty if the main earner can no longer work, as well as stress from caring and bereavement due to early deaths, To that, we can also add the stress caused to families today by having to pay hundreds of thousands of pounds for care in many cases, when this care would have been free when the NHS was originally set up, and until the 1970s. This pushes families under for several generations and leads to multigenerational health inequalities.

Looking at these issues in the round would help to determine:

(a) how these issues add up for individuals and families, and what is the full long-term health inequality impact
(b) what steps can be taken to make use of known ways to prevent death, for example reducing both outdoor and indoor pollution, improving housing, reducing stress, actively offering PGD IVF – a procedure which

identifies whether an embryo is affected by a serious genetic condition – to prevent genetic disease for future generations

(c) what steps can be taken to reduce the extra burden to individuals currently dying early, and their families, thanks to refusal of initial disability benefits claims, the loss of hardship grants for basic things like wheelchairs, charging huge care costs and preventing early claiming of state pensions. (These were all part of the original design of the welfare state so could definitely be afforded in the past, and far fewer people of working age are affected now.)

3. A new Beveridge Report

As John's story showed us, the Beveridge Report in the early 1940s was the natural follow-on from the TB inquiry in the late 1930s and built on its findings. Where the TB inquiry showed we needed a comprehensive health service and good quality housing, Beveridge suggested how this might be implemented in practice.

The Beveridge Report was particularly important because it showed how things had become fragmented. Many different organisations were supporting people in need. Some were giving wildly different levels of support to people with the same needs, and many people fell through the gaps and were not getting any support at all. Trying to sort all that out at a low level would take forever.

Instead, Beveridge proposed to turn things around and standardise provision of each service, such as health, housing and welfare benefits. Each service would be provided through one single national organization with local offices in each area. This immediately revolutionised efficiency and meant a standard level or service across the country, which was fairer for everyone. A new Beveridge Report today could look at how these services have been fragmented over time in the 75 years since the welfare state was established.

An example is the split between the NHS, social care and public health. In the original 1948 model, these essential services had been found by the TB inquiry to not work well when managed by local authorities, so they were all moved into the NHS. Then from the 1970s, some things started to be moved back to local authorities. This split has created a number of issues because all aspects of health, including prevention and care for people with medical conditions, are interlinked.

Could we look back at the original NHS and welfare state model in the Beveridge Report, to find better ways of doing this and replacing the current fragmented system with a more coordinated model? A new Beveridge Report could consider how people's needs are equitably met across the NHS and welfare state today, in particular looking at how people who are facing early death below age 65 are supported.

Beveridge also proposed setting benefits levels by looking at people's actual needs – a revolutionary concept at the time. What was the minimum level of income that people needed in order to live a healthy life? How much did the weekly food shopping and other essentials such as clothing, shoes and utilities cost for each size of family? How much did they need to pay for housing costs? Beveridge had found through research that most people have similar living costs in most parts of the country, with the exception of housing costs, which therefore need to be treated differently. Therefore housing costs should be based on people's actual housing costs. Other benefits should be based on an average cost.

Beveridge also made some very pertinent points about balancing supporting people in need with the need to avoid benefit fraud, as described by Chris Renwick in his study of the origins of the welfare state:

> There was also the question of what to do about people who did not pay into his proposed system? Surely universal benefits would be ripe for exploitation by some of these people?
>
> For centuries, critics of any attempt to understand poverty in terms of anything but individual character had painted apocalyptic scenes of huge numbers of feckless people milking the system. Such fevered imaginings had little to do with reality, as the experience of running social insurance since 1911 – not to mention the Poor Law before that – had shown.... While there were certainly people who were happy to take handouts rather than work, they were, Beveridge argued, in a small minority. There was no need to build a system around them and punish the rest of the population in the process.[2]

As at the time of the TB inquiry, housing is currently a key issue. It was solved in 1948 so could be solved again today, if we take a unified national approach. Beveridge made sure the government was directly in charge of new housebuilding – it was not farmed out to commercial developers to hope they would do the right thing, when this currently means more and more housebuilding in London and the south-east, with unaffordable rents and purchase prices. A government-led scheme could instead build social housing in strategic places and at controlled rents, making sure new infrastructure and jobs are also secured for each area.

We need a renewed understanding of why the whole welfare state is important, in order for the NHS to work effectively, and a return to optimum funding and organisation for each part.

As we have seen in great detail from the TB inquiry in the late 1930s, nearly everyone who has worked in health and social care for a long time knows full well that wicked problems like the Five Giants can only be resolved by tackling root causes. These include not only healthcare but also poverty, unemployment, housing, education, public health, prevention and self-management, and home care. It is nearly always cheaper to deal with the root cause than to pay for extra A&E staff to pick up the pieces. For example a decent minimum income level for everyone will resolve a lot of issues that currently crop up because people can't follow medical advice to eat healthily or follow a medically required diet.

4. Full death statistics on underlying causes of death
Full death statistics showing the underlying cause of death are essential to tackle the remaining causes of death below age 65 today. For example, pneumonia should not be the cause of death shown on the statistics, when the real cause of death is actually, say, a genetic disease like Huntington's.

All causes of death should be published even if only a small number of people die of that specific cause. This will help identify exact causes of death and bring together groups of similar conditions for research and treatment.

While there have been attempts made over recent years to better record actual causes of death-on-death certificates, this has not yet filtered through to the publicly available statistics. This is particularly the case for less common diseases, where only a small number of people in a local area die from that disease. This is on grounds of confidentiality. Yet as a person with a less common disease myself, I would be very happy to waive the confidentiality in order to help the NHS tackle my disease more effectively. After all, the statistics just show causes of death, not your name.

This will also help women with autoimmune conditions, known by scientific studies to be a current top ten cause of death in women, yet not recognized at all by the current death statistics. This has led to a lack of funding for this set of conditions, as would be warranted if it was clear to all NHS decision-makers and clinicians that these are such a common cause of death. As autoimmune conditions are hard to diagnose, if their doctor suspects the death may have resulted from an undiagnosed autoimmune condition, this should also be stated on the cause of death statistics.

It would also be helpful to include people who have suffered from trauma and people who are known or suspected to be on the autism spectrum, as these are both known to be causes of early death. If a person has committed suicide due to a disease, the disease should also be stated as the main cause of death rather than just suicide – the same with traffic accidents as these are sometimes disguised suicides of people with fatal diseases. Tracking the proper underlying cause using death statistics can therefore help to work out exactly what happens and how to help people more effectively in future.

5. Funding priority for people under 65 with fatal diseases
In recent years, it has been believed that equality meant everyone being given the same amount. This has now been superseded by an understanding that what we are actually aiming for is equity: everyone being given enough support to bring them into a fair situation which is equitable with others. The classic cartoon about equity shows three people of different heights all wanting to watch an event. One person can already see over the fence, so they do not need any support. The second person is just a little too short to see over the fence, so they need to stand on a small box, i.e. have a small amount of support. The third person is shorter, so needs to stand on a larger box, i.e., have a larger amount of support. Now all three people are on a level where they can see the event and are therefore in an equitable position.

The push in the late 1930s was to help people under 65 with fatal diseases as the NHS's highest priority. Due to age discrimination legislation, this appears to have been interpreted that younger people can no longer be prioritised for support and treatment. This is because it is thought that older people should have a right to the same care and treatment. This is not equitable for younger people because the older person has already enjoyed more healthy years of life than they have. Equitable use of resources therefore means that the priority should be to get everyone to age 65 with no major health issues.

Another key issue with equity for younger adults at the moment is differential treatment between diseases. If I had cancer, which these days is often not fatal, I would enjoy completely free treatment and home care from the NHS, and support services from large cancer charities, and, if I was to die, full pain relief. Instead, as I have a fatal genetic disease there is little than can be done medically for me so I fall through the funding gaps, which has major knock-on effects for me, and for my family.

6. Experts by Experience as a paid career

In recent years, the use of Experts by Experience has grown rapidly in the NHS and this is a very positive step.[3] Experts by Experience are people who have diseases themselves, and therefore know what it is like to use NHS services. As one person often has care from multiple different services, it is tricky for a clinician in one service to see things from the service user or patient perspective.

As Experts by Experience we often know instinctively where there is wasted effort in the system and can help overcome this. For example, I know that having a vast number of hospital appointments for my secondary autoimmune conditions has not been useful. This is in terms of my time, the hospital doctor's, and the poor old GP who has to keep on referring and re-referring, as the hospital has waiting list targets and even if your condition is not diagnosed you have to go back on the waiting list for the next hospital appointment so that you don't mess up the target by having a tricky-to-diagnose condition. This process could be made far simpler and cheaper by, for example, a detailed online symptom questionnaire which then suggests what to try next. This can include both things that the doctor has to do, like a urine test for diabetes, and things that the patient can try themselves while on the waiting list, like ruling out different triggers such as food groups.

The biggest issue I have found with using my experience in this way is that it is not paid. As I have bills to pay (like most people, even those of us with disabilities) this means I have to do other paid work as my main activity and therefore can only contribute to Experts by Experience work piecemeal, as a volunteer. I cannot work in detail on a project to really get into root causes and work with people to solve them.

At present, there have only started to be a few jobs for Experts by Experience and these tend to be only for mental health trusts, for people who have experienced mental health issues. Creating Experts by Experience paid roles for people with physical health conditions too would be a huge step forward. The current Experts By Experience roles are only junior peer support roles with one of the lowest salary levels in the NHS, with no input into higher level policy or decision-making. If we are really serious about the value of Experts by Experience, this should be a career pathway including all grades, based on what the person would get paid for other work in the NHS. Longer-term, entry-level Experts by Experience should be offered full training including civil service fast stream and equivalent, to ensure people with lived experience can be promoted to the highest levels in the NHS.

7. Teaching people about radical administration

For people to change the world today, we need to understand the key concepts of radical administration used by John Tomley and other changemakers. Systems thinking is now starting to be taught to a few primary school children, for example through the newly formed Ministry of Eco Education set up by Ecotricity, yet most children and adults are not yet trained in this approach. The other concepts – the social determinants of health, big data, and other useful social change tools such as theory of change – are not widely known either. These are the key tools we have to change our world, solve the health and social care crisis and solve the environmental crisis.

There is plenty of information available to us on these subjects, but how do we capture people's attention?

One way is to package these linked concepts into a whole, so that people can realise they are linked and easily refer to them. That's why I have called them 'radical administration', as it clearly links to how John worked, using what looked like normal administration tasks yet reframing them in a new, radical way to change the course of history. The exact name we use doesn't really matter of course. What matters is easily being able to get these tools out there, and a snappy and interesting sounding name which makes people curious to learn more.

An easy way to start off is to add these concepts to the National Curriculum at both primary and secondary school level. That will start off children and young people learning about these ways of working and telling their parents. Wales has already taken a lead here, which England and Scotland could follow: a new Curriculum for Wales was launched in 2022 which includes systems thinking.[4]

We also need to cover these concepts in depth in professional training courses for new health and social care workers doing qualifications in medicine, nursing, social care, public health and so on, as well as NHS and civil service management and administration trainees. Teaching all trainee accountants, lawyers, and management consultants too will help the concepts travel further across all sectors, from the charity sector to the

NHS, to the rest of the public sector, to business, and back again, with added improvements developed over time. Over time, newly qualified young people in workplaces will then be able to use these concepts. Over perhaps 20 years, these young people will end up in decision-making roles and be able to put these concepts into practice on a large scale.

Yet the health and social care crisis and the environmental crisis can't wait 20 years for this type of new knowledge to trickle down. So we must also roll out professional, free short courses online to cover everyone currently in work, so that people already at mid-career in positions of influence now, and their colleagues, can hear about these powerful tools and start to use them to tackle the issues we face today, together.

Endnotes

Opening Quotations

1. *Daily Herald*, 23 March 1939
2. William Beveridge, *Social Insurance and Allied Services*, 1942.
3. National Library of Wales, NRA Code:GB 0210 WNMA

Introduction: The Five Giants

1. Lady Charlotte Guest, *The Mabinogion, Translated from the Red Book of Hergest*, 1838
2. William Beveridge, *Social Insurance and Allied Services*, 1942.

Chapter 1: 'Merits Rarely Combined': 1872–1905

1. J. D. K. Lloyd, *A Montgomery Notebook*, 1971
2. *Y Genedl Gymreig*, 6 Mehefin (June) 1888
3. From John Tomley's personal letters held by his family.
4. Lloyd, *Notebook*
5. Ibid.
6. Ibid.
7. J. E. Tomley, *The Castle of Montgomery*, c.1930s
8. Lloyd, *Notebook*
9. *The Montgomery County Times*, 9 December 1893
10. *Montgomeryshire Express and Radnor Times*, 23 March 1892
11. J. D. K. Lloyd, *A Montgomery Notebook*, 1971
12. *Oddfellows Magazine*, Jul-Sep 1941
13. *Montgomeryshire Express and Radnor Times*, 23 June 1891
14. https://www.oddfellows.co.uk/about/traditions/
15. https://libcom.org/article/secret-handshakes-and-health-care-australia
16. *Montgomeryshire Express and Radnor Times*, 3 November 1891
17. Angus Snow, *John Dillon Snow 1886-1958*, 2006

18. N. Thomas-Symonds, *NYE: The Political Life of Aneurin Bevan*, 2014
19. *Montgomeryshire Express and Radnor Times*, 23 August 1892
20. *The Montgomery County Times*, 12 May 1894
21. *Montgomeryshire Express and Radnor Times*, 6 September 1892
22. *The Montgomery County Times*, 8 July 1893
23. *The Montgomery County Times*, 22 July 1893
24. *The Montgomery County Times*, 12 May 1894
25. Lloyd, *Notebook*
26. *The Montgomery County Times*, 19 August 1893
27. *The Montgomery County Times*, 3 February 1894
28. *The Wrexham Advertiser*, 3 February 1894
29. *Oddfellows Magazine*, Apr-Jun 1894
30. *Oswestry and Border Counties Advertizer*, 13 July 1892
31. *Oddfellows Magazine*, May-Aug 1901
32. *The Wellington Journal and Shrewsbury News*, 10 May 1902

Chapter 2: 'An Antidote to Pauperism': 1906–1911

1. *Oddfellows Magazine*, Jan-Apr 1905
2. *Oddfellows Magazine*, Jan-Apr 1903
3. *Border Counties Advertizer* – 14 Feb 1906
4. Ibid.
5. *The Manchester Guardian*, 4 April 1906
6. *The Manchester Guardian*, 9 May 1906
7. *Oddfellows Magazine*, Jul-Sep 1906
8. *The Staffordshire Sentinel*, 17 October 1908
9. *The Shrewsbury Chronicle*, 4 December 1908
10. *Oddfellows Magazine*, May-Aug 1909
11. *Oddfellows Magazine*, May-Aug 1910
12. Lloyd, *Notebook*
13. *The Montgomeryshire Express and Radnor Times*, 4 December 1906
14. https://viewer.library.wales/4683286#?xywh=438%2C1269%2C2891%2C3188&cv=65
15. https://viewer.library.wales/4683286#?xywh=357%2C2371%2C3219%2C3550&cv=66
16. *The Welsh Gazette*, 22 September 1910
17. https://www.independent.co.uk/news/health/nhs-70th-anniversary-founding-labour-aneurin-bevan-clement-attlee-welfare-state-british-history-a8407471.html

18. *The Barmouth County Advertiser and District Weekly News*, 29 September 1910.
19. W. H. Auden, *Spain,* 1937
20. *Hamilton Advertiser*, 15 October 1910
21. *Oddfellows Magazine*, May-Aug 1911
22. *Oddfellows Magazine*, Sep-Dec 1911

Chapter 3: 'Enough to Keep Body and Soul Alive': 1912–1922

1. *Oddfellows Magazine*, May-Aug 1912
2. *Oddfellows Magazine*, May-Aug 1912
3. *The Welsh Gazette*, 22 February 1912
4. https://viewer.library.wales/4683286#?xywh=555%2C803%2C2897%2C3195&cv=86
5. *The Liverpool Daily Post and Mercury,* 30 July 1912
6. *Nottingham Evening Post*, 27 September 1912
7. *Oddfellows Magazine*, Sep-Dec 1912
8. *Oddfellows Magazine*, Jul 1914
9. Ibid.
10. Ibid.
11. Ibid.
12. *Oddfellows Magazine*, Oct-Dec 1913
13. *Oddfellows Magazine*, May-Aug 1912
14. *Oddfellows Magazine*, Jan-Mar 1913
15. *Oddfellows Magazine*, Apr-May 1913
16. Ibid.
17. *Oddfellows Magazine*, Jun 1913
18. *Oddfellows Magazine*, Jul 1914
19. *County Times*, 2 December 1922
20. https://www.kingsfund.org.uk/blog/2017/02/funding-health-care-great-war
21. *County Times*, 2 December 1922
22. *Oddfellows Magazine*, Mar-Apr 1915
23. *Oddfellows Magazine*, Sep-Dec 1915
24. *County Times*, 2 December 1922
25. *Oddfellows Magazine*, Sep-Dec 1916
26. Parliamentary papers, *Old age pensions: Appendix to the report of the Departmental Committee on Old Age Pensions, including minutes of evidence,* 1919

27. *Oddfellows Magazine*, Jan-Apr 1920
28. *The Yorkshire Post*, 19 September 1919
29. *Oddfellows Magazine*, Oct-Nov 1919
30. Ibid.
31. https://viewer.library.wales/4683286#?xywh=128%
    2C978%2C3477%2C3834&cv=154
32. *Western Mail*, 31 October 1919
33. *The Story of Montgomery*, Ann & John Welton, 2003
34. https://viewer.library.wales/4683286#?xywh=504%2C2273%
    2C2891%2C3188&cv=171
35. *Oddfellows Magazine*, Aug-Dec 1921
36. Ibid.
37. *Oddfellows Magazine*, May-Jun 1920
38. *Oddfellows Magazine*, Jul 1922
39. *Liverpool Daily Post and Mercury*, 10 February 1922
40. *County Times*, 2 December 1922
41. *Oddfellows Magazine*, Aug-Dec 1922

Chapter 4: 'The Busy Man': 1923–1930

1. *Western Mail*, 13 June 1923
2. *Oddfellows Magazine*, Jan-Apr 1923
3. *Oddfellows Magazine*, Aug-Dec 1923
4. *The Yorkshire Post*, 10 June 1924
5. *The Devon and Exeter Gazette*, 14 June 1924
6. *Oddfellows Magazine*, Jul 1924
7. *Oddfellows Magazine*, Aug-Dec 1924
8. Pamela Michael & Charles Webster, *Health and Society in Twentieth-Century Wales*, 2006
9. Ibid.
10. *Oddfellows Magazine*, Jan-Apr 1924
11. *Oddfellows Magazine*, Aug 1925
12. *Oddfellows Magazine*, Jan-Mar 1926
13. https://www.wcia.org.uk/wcia-news/wcia-history/david-davies-75-father-of-the-temple-of-peace/
14. *Oddfellows Magazine*, Jul 1926
15. *Oddfellows Magazine*, Sep-Nov 1926
16. *The Yorkshire Post*, 9 June 1927
17. *Oddfellows Magazine*, May-Jun 1928

18. *Oddfellows Magazine*, Aug-Sep 1928
19. *Oddfellows Magazine*, Oct-Dec 1928
20. *Oddfellows Magazine*, Jul 1929
21. *Oddfellows Magazine*, Jul 1930
22. *Oddfellows Magazine*, Oct-Dec 1930
23. *Oddfellows Magazine*, Jan-Apr 1925
24. *Welsh Gazette*, 14 July 1927
25. *Merthyr Express*, 8 October 1927
26. *Western Mail*, 20 January 1930
27. *Western Mail & South Wales News*, 22 March 1930
28. *Welsh Gazette*, 29 January 1925
29. *Welsh Gazette*, 6 August 1925
30. *Western Mail*, 31 July 1926
31. *Welsh Gazette*, 8 November 1928
32. *Oddfellows Magazine*, Jan-Apr 1930
33. *Welsh Outlook*, 1930

Chapter 5: 'An Inquiry in My Own Way': 1931–1937

1. *Western Mail & South Wales News*, 28 September 1934
2. *Oddfellows Magazine*, Apr 1932
3. *Lincolnshire Standard*, 30 May 1931
4. *Oddfellows Magazine*, Oct 1931
5. *Oddfellows Magazine*, Jul 1932
6. *Oddfellows Magazine*, Oct 1932
7. *Oddfellows Magazine*, Sep-Oct 1933
8. *Oddfellows Magazine*, Mar-Apr 1934
9. *Oddfellows Magazine*, Jul 1934
10. *Oddfellows Magazine*, Oct-Dec 1934
11. Ibid.
12. *Western Mail & South Wales News*, 14 November 1931
13. *The Scotsman*, 15 July 1933
14. *Oddfellows Magazine*, Oct-Dec 1934
15. *Oddfellows Magazine*, Jan 1933
16. *Oddfellows Magazine*, May-Jun 1935
17. *Oddfellows Magazine*, Jul-Sep 1939
18. *Western Mail & South Wales News*, 3 August 1935
19. The National Archives, Kew – Ministry of Health MH55/1121 & MH 55/1215

20. *Oddfellows Magazine*, Jul-Sep 1939
21. *Sir William Beveridge, Social Insurance and Allied Services,* 1942
22. *Oddfellows Magazine*, Jul-Sep 1939
23. *Oddfellows Magazine*, Jul 1936
24. G. Goodwin, *Call Back Yesterday*, 1935
25. *Oddfellows Magazine*, Oct-Dec 1935
26. *Western Mail & South Wales News*, 8 May 1936
27. *Yorkshire Post and Leeds Intelligencer*, 4 June 1936
28. National Library of Wales, NRA Code: GB 0210 WNMA
29. *Western Mail & South Wales News*, 31 July 1936
30. *Western Mail & South Wales News*, 12 August 1936
31. *Western Mail & South Wales News*, 18 September 1936
32. *Oddfellows Magazine*, Jul-Sep 1939
33. Western Mail & South Wales News, 30 January 1937
34. The National Archives, Kew – Ministry of Health MH55/1121 & MH 55/1215
35. *Oddfellows Magazine*, Jul-Sep 1939

Chapter 6: 'No Mean Responsibility': 1937–1939

1. The Scotsman, 18 September 1937
2. *Western Mail & South Wales News*, 21 September 1937
3. *Western Mail & South Wales News*, 28 October 1937
4. *Western Mail & South Wales News*, 5 November 1937
5. *Oddfellows Magazine*, Jul-Sep 1939
6. The National Archives, Kew – Ministry of Health MH55/1121 & MH 55/1215
7. https://www.wcia.org.uk/wcia-news/wcia-history/david-davies-75-father-of-the-temple-of-peace/
8. The National Archives, Kew – Ministry of Health MH55/1121 & MH 55/1215
9. *Western Mail & South Wales News*, 19 January 1938
10. *Oddfellows Magazine*, Jul-Sep 1939
11. *Oddfellows Magazine*, Oct-Dec 1938
12. *Oddfellows Magazine*, Oct-Dec 1938
13. https://lloydgeorgesociety.org.uk/en/document/clement-davies-triumph-and-tragedy-a-personal-portrait-of-the-former-liberal-leader.pdf
14. *Oddfellows Magazine*, Jan-Mar 1939

15. Clement Davies MP & Dr F. J. H Coutts, Report of the Committee of Inquiry into the Anti-Tuberculosis Service in Wales, 1937-39
16. *Daily Mirror*, 14 March 1939
17. *Daily Sketch*, 14 March 1939
18. *Western Mail & South Wales News*, 16 March 1939
19. *Sunday Graphic and Sunday News*, 19 March 1939
20. Hansard, *HC Deb 22 March 1939 vol 345 cc1330-421*
21. *Daily Herald*, 23 March 1939
22. *Oddfellows Magazine*, Apr-Jun 1939
23. *Oddfellows Magazine*, Jul-Sep 1939
24. *Oddfellows Magazine*, Jul-Sep 1939
25. *Oddfellows Magazine*, Oct-Dec 1939

Chapter 7: 'The Unknown Friend': 1940–1951

1. Lloyd, *Notebook*
2. *Oddfellows Magazine*, Apr-Jun 1940
3. *Oddfellows Magazine*, Jul-Sep 1941
4. *Oddfellows Magazine*, Jul-Dec 1943
5. https://lloydgeorgesociety.org.uk/en/document/clement-davies-triumph-and-tragedy-a-personal-portrait-of-the-former-liberal-leader.pdf
6. *Western Mail & South Wales News*, 27 April 1943
7. *Oddfellows Magazine*, Jan-Jun 1943
8. *Western Mail & South Wales News*, 15 September 1943
9. *Oddfellows Magazine*, Jan-Jun 1945
10. https://archive.org/details/reportssubmitted1931univ
11. *Oddfellows Magazine*, Jul-Dec 1945
12. National Library of Wales, NRA Code: GB 0210 WNMA
13. *Oddfellows Magazine*, Mar-Apr 1946
14. *Western Mail & South Wales News*, 18 October 1946
15. National Library of Wales, NRA Code: GB 0210 WNMA
16. National Library of Wales, NRA Code: GB 0210 WNMA
17. *County Times*, 31 July 1948
18. *Oddfellows Magazine*, Nov-Dec 1948
19. *Oddfellows Magazine*, Dec 1949
20. *Oddfellows Magazine*, Nov 1950
21. *Oddfellows Magazine*, Nov 1950
22. *Oddfellows Magazine*, Jul-Sep 1951
23. *Oddfellows Magazine*, May 1962

Epilogue: After John

1. Adam Kay, *This is Going to Hurt: Secret Diaries of a Junior Doctor*, 2017
2. https://hansard.parliament.uk/Commons/1969-04-23/debates/24a813cf-67c5-4479-89ed-c2e55a2e5e60/SheltonHospital
3. https://www.shropshirestar.com/news/nostalgia/2018/02/28/deadly-fire-which-changed-thinking-forever/

Afterword: The Five Giants Today

1. Mortality statistics, https://www.nomisweb.co.uk/
2. Chris Renwick, *Bread for All: The Origins of the Welfare State*, 2017
3. See https://www.cqc.org.uk/about-us/jobs/experts-experience
4. https://hwb.gov.wales/curriculum-for-wales/science-and-technology/statements-of-what-matters/